LJB X

3D

by Carol Showalter

and the **3D** Program

DIET

DISCIPLINE

& DISCIPLESHIP

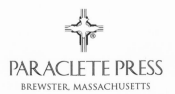

PARACLETE PRESS
BREWSTER, MASSACHUSETTS

Library of Congress Cataloging-in-Publication Data

Showalter, Carol.
    3D : diet, discipline & discipleship / Carol Showalter.—[New, rev. ed.].
        p. cm.
    ISBN 1-55725-294-7
    1. Showalter, Carol. 2. Diet, Discipline, and Discipleship, Inc. 3. Weight loss—Religious aspects—Christianity. 4. Reducing diets—Recipes. I. Title.
BX9225.S43 A35 2002
248.8'4—dc21   2001054554

ISBN: 1-55725-294-7

Published by Paraclete Press
Brewster, Massachusetts
www.paracletepress.com

Printed in the United States of America.

10 9 8 7 6 5 4 3 2 1

Thank you, Lord,

for your patience and love to me

as I respond to your call

in my life.

Thank you, family and friends—

you have always loved me and

encouraged me in that call.

Special gratitude to God for

David, Lillian, and M. Betty—

who knew God was able to do

exceedingly more than I could think

or imagine was possible!

CONTENTS

3D: The Story

3D: The Program

3D
The Story

by Carol Showalter

FOREWORD

My late mother-in-law was a godly woman. She was also much given to running, albeit insightful, commentary on the ways of the world and, most particularly, of the humanity around her. These sometimes piercing insights she rendered up in the Scotch-Irish near-brogue of the Tennessee mountains from which she came and in which she lived out her entire life.

In addition to being insightful, Mamaw's assessments were inevitably colorful. At times, they were almost parabolic, in fact; for she drew her wisdom from the natural well of many years on the land and many years of walking with her Lord in candid, rather than theoretical, prayer. And whatever else may be said of her, it must also be said that she would have understood Carol Showalter immediately. She would also have approved.

(My suspicion, for what it's worth, is that the reverse would also have been true, but that's a different issue. Suffice it to say here that I loved one of them ferociously and love the other completely, making a mutual affection between them seem entirely reasonable to me despite their separation in time, place, and circumstance.)

Mamaw's supply of observations and aphorismic stories was as rich and varied as her keen ear and sharp mind were accomplished; none the less, she had her favorites among them, ones which she took out, brushed off, and applied with regularity wherever appropriate. Her favorite amongst the tales was one about a middle-aged German farmer who had migrated from the old country up into the fertile Appalachian valleys near Mamaw's girlhood home. He had, she said, seven children, and he bought twelve acres of land on which to rear them. Unfortunately, she also said, he could not make a go of things on twelve acres; so being a wise man, he sold off ten acres and did quite nicely with feeding and rearing his brood on the remaining two acres to which he could at last pay close attention.

The wisdom here can be called—frequently is called, in fact—"mountain wisdom" or "folk wisdom." It is, of course, but it is also far more. It is spiritual wisdom. Specifically, it is called discipline and is remarkably hard to apply in the flat lands and among those of us who are today's urbanized, sophisticated folk. Carol Showalter knows that. It is part of what this book is about.

But what this book is also about has more to do with Mamaw's most telling, though rarely employed, observation than with her favorite fable. What she would upon occasion say was, "That man (or woman, as the case might be) has a fat soul."

On the few times I ever heard her speak those words about another human being, her tone of voice ranged somewhere between regret and outright sorrow. There clearly was neither condemnation nor even criticism in this most serious of assessments. Rather, there was a kind of spiritual diagnosis which took the metaphor of physical corpulence and applied it to the ill health of an undisciplined spirit. Carol Showalter understands that completely. So, too, do the thousands and thousands of men and women who, over the last twenty-seven years, have found in the 3D program and its three "D's" of diet, discipline, and discipleship a way to thin their souls and their bodies back to new life here and with their Lord. They have found, in other words, not only the courage and the methods, but a community of accountability that enables them . . . and Mamaw would have understood that.

So, welcome. Welcome to the company of many of your fellow Christians and welcome as well to the mentoring of one . . . I think two . . . very humble, very similar, and very wise women. May God bless and enrich every day of the journey that begins here.

Phyllis Tickle

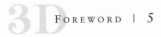

PREFACE

It would take literally hundreds of pages to share with you the life of the 3D program as it has existed from the end of the original story until now. Instead, I asked God to give you, through my own spiritual journey, the essence of the teaching of 3D and what it has continued to do in my own life and in the lives of everyone in the program.

Very little has changed from the beginning. God brought forth a program and put it all in place in the first 12 weeks. What God does He does well. I have carried the vision He gave me and the passion of knowing that His love and mercy are always at work in my life. I invite you to join me as I share these thoughts about the principles and power of this, the first Christian diet program.

I will then introduce you to wonderful friends from the past and the present who have been a part of 3D. We have journeyed together towards the same goal—to grow in our spiritual lives. And God has used 3D as part of that journey.

Many times in the past, people would finish the *3D* book, and their first question was, "What do I do next?" They would call our office and become informed about the program and the materials. In this new, revised edition of the book, everything you need to know will be right between these two covers. The diet will be explained, as well as the disciplines you are encouraged to participate in—exercise, prayer, Bible reading, journaling, and daily devotional readings. The only things missing from these pages are the daily readings you will need for spiritual growth, and I will tell you how to get your copy.

God be with you and bless you and cause you to grow in His love and mercy and compassion towards yourself and towards others.

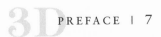

SMILE, GOD HAS THE ANSWER

"Tim, Betsy," I called, looking out the window. "Get your sweaters on; the bus has just turned the corner." The route of bus #139 took it down Pixley Road, which bordered our lot, and then around the block before stopping in front of our house. It was handy. The children didn't have to wait outside, as long as I kept watch out the kitchen window.

It was becoming a beautiful fall day. The sunlight filtering through the trees in our yard in suburban Rochester, New York, was changing that morning from dark and brisk to bright and warm. Trees surrounded our house, and the first dabs of orange and yellow were appearing on the tips of the leaves. I loved the fall; it reminded me of New England, where I was born and raised.

Pulling his sweater over his head, Tim grabbed his bag lunch from the counter and headed for the front door. "Hey!" I said. He returned quickly to brush my cheek with a kiss, and flash a cocky smile before disappearing out the front door. Tim was nine and a half and was in the fifth grade.

"Betsy!" I yelled, "You're going to miss the bus."

Unhurried footsteps indicated she was coming. I grabbed her sweater off the chair, put it on her, and propelled her towards the front door. The bus was stopping out front. "Here's your lunch—now hurry." I watched her climb on the bus, waved my final good-bye, and went back to the kitchen. My bus watch was over, but instead of finishing the dishes, I knelt on the chair, looking out the window again, this time at the church parking lot across the street.

I was startled when my husband Bill slipped his arm around me.

"Didn't mean to scare you," he said. "I just wanted to kiss you goodbye before heading over to church." He paused and looked at me. "Where are your thoughts this beautiful fall morning?"

"Oh, I don't know; just daydreaming, I guess."

"What's so inviting out there?" he asked, resting his hands on my shoulders and looking out the window. Reaching up, I put my hands on top of his and said, "Nothing, honey. I'm just nosey and wonder what's going on at church."

The moment the words came out, I felt guilty. I knew exactly what I was looking for, but I didn't want to tell him. Not yet. "Well, okay," was his response, and he leaned down and kissed me and headed out the side door. "Don't forget it's Monday," he said over his shoulder, "and the men meet in my office for lunch. I'll need a sandwich." "Sure, hon, I'll bring one over just before noon. Have a good day."

I turned back to the window and watched my husband walk across the yard, heading towards the stately, red brick, colonial church. Bill was the senior minister of the Parkminster Presbyterian Church, one of Rochester's rapidly growing young congregations, and our manse was directly across the street from the church. We had moved here three years ago, in September of 1969, from an inner-city parish in Bridgeport, Connecticut. I had loved Bridgeport and hated to move, but more and more I was feeling very comfortable and happy in Rochester.

My eyes were still fixed on the parking lot. In drove a big red station wagon and out stepped a big red-coated lady. A moment later, a blue compact car parked beside the wagon. Its door opened; a huge lady in a raincoat struggled to get out. More cars were pulling in, and more fat ladies were getting out, all clad in coats, though the weather only called for sweaters. I knew the reason from experience: Overweight people usually think a coat masks their true girth. My question of the morning was being answered right before my eyes: Weight Watchers was still meeting at our church on Monday mornings.

Now I had to face the next question: Should I march myself over there and join that group today?

Just before falling asleep last night, I had promised myself that if they were still meeting, I would join. It was easy to make that promise last night. I had overeaten again at supper and then snacked on chocolate chip cookies just before I went upstairs. I was uncomfortably full. But now this morning, I was gradually convincing myself that if I really tried again to cut back, I could do it all by myself. After all, I did resist that second piece of toast at breakfast. But then, breakfast never did turn me on that much, so I knew underneath I wasn't too victorious.

I refused to talk to anyone about it, even Bill, because I couldn't bear to admit that my weight was out of control again. Last night I had finally made up my mind, but now I was fighting the reality of having to join that parade of fat women marching into the church. After all, I certainly wasn't that fat! "Mommy?" My thoughts were interrupted by a tug at my arm. "Let's go to church," came this tiny voice. There stood my two-and-a-half-year-old son, Peter. The nursery at church, where babysitting was available daily, was one of his favorite places. He could always count on a good time, with lots of friends and lots of toys. "Okay, Peter Stephen, I guess it's time to go." His words pushed me over the brink of indecision where I had been teetering all morning. I sighed and stood up. "Where's your jacket?" I asked, looking down at his big hazel eyes full of excitement.

He ran towards the hall closet and pointed up to his little blue corduroy jacket. I slipped it on him and zipped it up. I started to reach for my beige sweater but decided instead to wear my navy raincoat.

As we walked across the backyard, I spotted my neighbor Mildred at her window. She always made it a point to greet the children when they were out in the yard or walking over to church. I picked Peter up and pointed to her. He smiled and waved his hand furiously. She's probably noticed I've been getting fat again, I thought. Would she guess that I was headed over to the Weight Watchers meeting at church? Were any of the other neighbors looking out at Peter and me? Good Lord, what's the matter with me today? I'm practically paranoid about this weight thing. You would think I was some obese thing waddling across the yard!

Weight obsessed me. Whether I was gaining or losing, I was thinking about it most of the time. In fact, that was the first thing I noticed about other people, so I guess I was convinced that that was the first thing they noticed about me. And I'd judged overweight people for years. I was pretty proud that I could lose weight quite successfully. But I never stopped to face the cold fact that I gained weight just as successfully every year.

A very fat woman was walking into the side door of the church ahead of Peter and me. She went upstairs and I went downstairs. Ultimately we were both going to end up in the same room, but I would delay that situation a few minutes longer. I stood around the nursery long enough to settle Peter and finally trudged upstairs.

Walking into the room killed me. Fat women were all over the place. Some were sitting down, gabbing away; others were in lines, waiting for one thing or another. Three women in the room, out of fifty or sixty, had decent figures. And two of these were sitting at the table, registering people for class.

The class was being held in what we called the East Hall. It used to be the sanctuary of the original church, which we had outgrown, but was now used for Sunday school classes and community groups such as this. It was a good, large room, with plenty of space for rows of chairs, tables for registrations, and a private weigh-in area. A number of partitions were shifted around the room to set off the particular needs of the program. I took my place in the line of women waiting to register.

This weight battle had been going on in my life for such a long time—over ten years. In the course of a year I would gain twenty or twenty-five pounds, and then in two or three months I would lose them any way I could. I had tried all kinds of crash diet programs that sometimes worked and sometimes didn't. I would eat only one thing for three or four weeks and usually lose the weight pretty quickly. (I remember one time eating only beets for three weeks!) But the least painful method for me, or so I thought, was to take diet pills— prescribed amphetamines—which the teenagers called "speed."

They certainly took my desire for food away, but at the same time I would also lose close touch with reality. Talking too much and flitting nervously from one thing to another was usually a sure sign that I was into the bottle of pills again. But if Bill would question me at all, I would squirm around the subject. "You seem awfully hyper to me," he would say. "Are you taking those darn diet pills again?" "Why do you always blame the diet pills?" I would respond. "The real problem with me is that there is too much work that has to be done at church and around the house. Maybe if you'd get me some more help in those areas, I wouldn't be so hyper!"

That would usually cow him, and he wouldn't say any more. And I would continue to take the diet pills, until the amount of weight I had to lose was gone. This went on for at least four years. Bill did not dare say much, but I knew he was alarmed that I was so dependent on diet pills. And in the late sixties, the drug scene was getting pretty bad. I finally decided I shouldn't have those pills around the house with teenage babysitters and church groups over so often, so I flushed what I had down the toilet, vowing never to use them again. Naturally, I waited to do this until I was thin again.

Now, with the diet pills gone, and the crash diets growing less and less successful as I grew older, I knew I had to find another route to get rid of my excess weight each year. In May 1970 I went to see my doctor for my yearly checkup. "Mrs. Showalter?" I put my magazine down and stood up to follow a nurse with a clipboard in her hand. "Would you come this way, please?" I followed closely behind her, trying to be amiable, but she was all business. "Beautiful day, isn't it?" I suggested. No response.

She stopped abruptly at the gray monster—the hospital scale outside the doctor's office. "Please step up here, so I can check your weight for the doctor." I started to take off my shoes, but she said, "That isn't necessary, Mrs. Showalter, it won't make much difference." Well, I knew she was wrong! Shoes do make a difference, and so does the time of day and several other things, but there was no sense in arguing with her. I'd just deduct in my own mind what I thought those shoes weighed and also a pound or so because it was the middle of the afternoon, and I always weighed more at that time.

The bottom weight indicator was set in the 100-pound notch. She pushed the top weight to the far right. Nothing happened; the balance bar at the end of the scale cleaved to the top—147, 148, 150, still nothing. "Looks like we'll have to move up a notch," she remarked casually. That meant into the 150-pound notch. If only she had let me take off my shoes.

The clunk of the weight as she changed it seemed to echo all over the waiting room. I was sure everyone heard it for a mile around.

She kept moving the top weight, but still nothing happened. My eyes were glued to the balance bar; when would it detach itself from the top? Oh, no, 160, 165, and now finally a slight movement, and slowly it began to descend. I was 167½ pounds and devastated. I expected that I would be over 150, but never did I dream I was back up there—again.

My doctor was angry when he read the chart. "Get that weight off, Carol, and quickly! You're too young to weigh almost 170 pounds." I didn't say anything, but inside I was furious. Who did he think he was? I was there for my gynecological checkup, not a lecture on weight control. "As soon as you leave here today, I want you to find the diet group nearest to your house and join it right away. Like Weight Watchers or Diet Workshop. Either of those near you?"

I dearly wished I could have lied at that point. But I paused and gulped noticeably, "Yes, Weight Watchers has two groups that meet in our church every week." "Well, there can't be anything more convenient," he smiled. But he wouldn't just drop it. He went on to talk about how young mothers fall into depression from being overweight, and how older people literally die from overweight, and on and on.

I was insulted and angry, but his confrontation worked. The next week I joined Weight Watchers. (To my chagrin I weighed in at 167 lbs. that first meeting—without my shoes and before breakfast!) And the program worked for me. The first twenty pounds went quickly, and then I got comfortable and lazy for a while. I thought I looked pretty good at 147, and I was not as anxious to get the rest off. In fact it wasn't until August 1971, fifteen months after I joined, that I graduated at 130 pounds. Naturally, I was totally convinced that I would never, never gain weight again. Finally, I knew how and what to eat. It would be easy from here on—or so I thought.

Now, in October 1972, I was standing in line at the same Weight Watchers group, waiting to register again. The line had been moving steadily, and I was facing the thin registration clerk. She told me to fill out the front and back questions on the payment book and said the weekly fee was $2.50, in addition to a $5.00 registration fee. "Does it make any difference that I'm a graduate of this program?" I asked quietly. (I never would have mentioned it, but I had a hunch the cost was less for ex-members.) "Oh," she said, looking up at me, perhaps trying to remember my face. "Do you have your lifetime membership book with you?" "No, I'm sorry, and I haven't the vaguest idea what I did with it. I hadn't planned on using it again," I mumbled.

I hated the humiliation of needing Weight Watchers, and its membership certificate was not something I treasured. I had buried it somewhere and quickly forgotten about it. "I'll look in our files and see if we have your old registration number and weight chart, Mrs. Showalter. In the meantime, why don't you just step over to the other line and wait to be weighed in."

The line I was now in was moving towards one of the room dividers. There were voices behind the divider, but the conversations were not discernible. "Next, please," were the only words that clearly came over the top of the partition. While I was still standing there, the clerk brought me my new book. "You don't have to pay the registration fee, Mrs. Showalter," she said, handing me back a five-dollar bill. "And if, I mean, when, you get within two pounds of your goal, you will no longer have to pay the weekly fee, either. Those are the privileges of our graduates," she said, smiling and giving a plug for the program to those within earshot.

As I waited in line, I began to wonder where that membership book could be . . . probably with the tiny square box that said "Congratulations" on the front of it. Inside was a silver pin, with diamond chips, indicating that I was a successful graduate of the program. I never wore the pin. I wasn't about to advertise the fact that I was ever fat!

Soon the "Next, please" was for me. I stepped behind the divider and handed my book to a slender, gray-haired woman. She didn't even bother to look up. I was only a number to her. "Step on the scale, please." "Can't I take off my shoes?" I pleaded. "Of course," she answered, as if I should have known better than to ask. She was obviously in a hurry. There were still a dozen women behind me, waiting to be weighed.

Things hadn't changed much in the past two years. The weigher could read the weight, but the person on the scale had the numbers blocked by a large, strategically placed, piece of cardboard with a "fat" joke on it.

That had always irritated me, because I wanted to know what I weighed—exactly. And I didn't trust her honesty. Besides, why should she know my weight, before I knew it? Whose body was it anyway? "You're 147½, Mrs. Showalter," she announced. "That's a relief! I was sure I'd be over 150," I said, trying to cheer myself up. "Well," she replied, smiling, "it wasn't that long ago you were 130 pounds, was it?"

I groaned. How did she know? It probably was written in that exasperating little lifetime membership book. I picked up my payment book and headed out. The next lady was already behind the partition, taking off her shoes.

Choosing a seat on the end of the very last row, I noticed that the only man in the room was at the other end—a very big, fat man, reading a newspaper. Actually, he did not appear to be interested in the paper, but he seemed even less interested in talking to any of the women in the hall. I felt the same way. I too, preferred to do my socializing elsewhere. Unfortunately, I didn't have a newspaper or anything else to read, so I had to find some other way to avoid conversations. I began to look around the room for objects of interest. Bible verses were written on blackboards, and Sunday school papers were tacked up on the various partitions. One partition caught my attention: a big, red smile face was painted right on the rough finish of the partition. The face was trimmed widely with black paint and there were large bold words beside it: *Smile, God Has The Answer.*

I couldn't take my eyes off those words. Smile—I wasn't in the mood. "If God has the answer, why am I here?" I asked myself. "I feel miserable sitting in this room. But I have to get this weight off again, before I climb back up to 170." And I knew very well I was on my way; I could feel it.

That smile sign was disgustingly persistent. It made me mad. I knew God has answers for lots of problems, but He had never helped me with my weight problem! Yes, answers for searching teenagers, answers for troubled marriages, answers for big problems, but. . . .

I squirmed. Hey, preacher's wife, won't your God help you? Can't you practice what you preach to so many others? The thoughts coming at me from the potent sign were like poison darts.

But I *had* prayed. Many, many nights I had prayed. Falling asleep, I would beg God to please take away my desire for the fattening S's—sweets, snacks, and seconds! But I would wake up and hardly be able to wait until breakfast to take the first bite of a doughnut. Then after breakfast, I'd remember God and throw up a quick prayer, asking Him to keep all temptations away from me throughout the day, quickly quoting the verse in 1 Corinthians that said, "There has no temptation overtaken you but such as is common to man. But God is faithful and just and will not allow you to be tempted above that which you are able to bear. . . ." Now it was up to God to just keep those temptations away from me. The responsibility was on Him. But I would bump smack into moist chocolate chip cookies, sticky sweet rolls, and filled candy dishes everywhere I turned. I couldn't resist! "If only He had kept the temptations away," I would say to myself, enjoying every bite of my "sin." I was still looking at the smile face, when a voice up front interrupted my thoughts. "Good morning, ladies! And to our newcomers, welcome to Weight Watchers! We have been meeting here at Parkminster Church for over two years now, and every week we add new members."

The speaker was an attractive woman of about thirty-five. I had seen her buzzing around the room and assumed that she was the lecturer. She had the best figure in the room, and the way she was dressed and strutted around, it was obvious that it was a relatively new figure of which she was proud.

I was jealous of it. "Before we get too far into today's meeting," she went on, "I have something for you to see—a picture of me three summers ago." She flashed an enlarged picture of herself draped over a chaise lounge eating a piece of cake and drinking something out of a can. The fat was literally hanging off of her lifted arm, and she was bulging over the sides of the lounge. It was hard to believe that it was really her. "I've lost 106 pounds and have kept just about all of it off for almost three years now. And if I can do it, so can you!"

It was a good thing she said, "just about all of it," because I could see at least ten pounds that she shouldn't be carrying.

I looked around the room; her audience was dazzled. Those fat ladies were hungrily picturing themselves standing up front a year from now, a trim size twelve. You could see the dreams in their eyes. For the next ten minutes, she talked about the emotional and medical dangers for fat people, emphasizing her points with a hand-made flip chart, full of statistics. I was bored and tuned her out. That smile face was still grinning at me, and I was pouting back at it.

Suddenly the thought struck me: Was God trying to say something to me through that sign? Perhaps half an hour had passed since I first had seen that big red face and those five words. Maybe God had an answer for me I hadn't heard before. I had no idea what it could be. The lecturer continued. Names were being called now, and an announcement of how much weight each person had lost in the week. There was laughter and clapping after each name, but I was not a part of it. I was busy making a decision. "All new members must stay after the class for a few minutes, so that I can explain some of the details of the diet," she said, pointing to the side of the room I was sitting on. "We'll meet over there. The rest of you are free to go now. Have a good week, everyone," she said, waving goodbye.

While the majority of the ladies headed towards the door, six or seven were making their way to the rows she had pointed to. I got up and headed for the door myself. I could almost feel the lecturer's eyes on my back. At that moment I had no idea what I was going to do about my weight problem after I walked out that door. But I knew God was going to help me—somehow. He did have the answer. And as I slipped out the door, just before it closed, I was almost smiling.

I picked up Peter in the nursery, and we walked back across the parking lot and the yard to the house. I felt peaceful now. And I began to see some things about myself. I had to stop putting the blame on God for not answering my prayers. The problem was me, not God. I loved to eat—I just hated to gain weight. And even after "willing" the weight off through Weight Watchers, I still chose to begin eating the wrong foods again. And no amount of praying in the morning or at night was going to magically wash those calories away. If I ate what I wanted, when I wanted to, I was going to get fat again. It was as simple as that. The problem was not God, nor was it with the Weight Watchers program. The problem was me! And it was about time I faced that.

As soon as we walked in the kitchen door, Peter interrupted those thoughts mulling around in my head. "Can I have a cookie, Mommy?" he asked, pointing up to the cookie jar. "Sure, Tiger," and I got one out for him—just one.

THE END OF A PRETEND WORLD

In the months that followed that October morning in 1972, I found that my weight problem no longer consumed my thoughts, yet at the same time I didn't try to avoid it. It seemed like the whole thing was simply de-emphasized. I was still heavier than I should have been, but I was peaceful. And something else: The compulsive eating seemed to stop. I wasn't losing, but I wasn't gaining, either. And I was able to hold it around 145 pounds.

Almost before I knew it, fall and winter had passed, and spring was upon us. Spring is a time of celebration for upstate New Yorkers. The intensely cold winters are a full five months long, and the first signs of spring are welcomed jubilantly with, among other things, the planning of a spring luncheon at church. So when the first buds appeared on the lilac trees, and tulips and daffodils began to push their noses through the ground, the women of the church began to plan their annual spring luncheon. The date this year would be May 3rd.

The table decorations would be as many different colors of spring flowers as could be found in the early gardens, and women from all over the community would be invited. The guest speakers were two women who were not strangers to our congregation, Mrs. Cay Andersen and Mrs. Judy Sorensen.

Bill and I had first heard Cay and Judy, as they were popularly known, twelve years earlier, in 1961, at a Faith at Work conference in Northfield, Massachusetts. They had shared how God had called them, in a little church on Cape Cod, to minister together as a team, counseling and leading retreats at various churches around New England.

Cay's husband, Bill, was a builder, and they owned and operated a beautiful guesthouse at Rock Harbor, near Orleans, with their son, Peter. They led a relatively peaceful life. Although Cay had been a very sick woman for several years, she was now able to manage the guesthouse. The Sorensen family, Judy and Bill, who was a business executive, and their four children, vacationed on Cape Cod every year. Before long, the Sorensens moved in with the Andersens at Rock Harbor—four adults and five children under one roof. The teaching they had done at Northfield and at other churches was based largely on the experiences they were having in living out the Christian life under these circumstances (long before community living had gained any popular acceptance).

Our first reaction to their sharing was mixed. Bill was put off by their lack of formal Christian training, and yet they intrigued him. "They're so spontaneous!" I exclaimed. "They don't seem to prepare their talks, and they don't seem to know who is going to speak first or say what." We came away not quite knowing what to make of these two ladies from Cape Cod.

Then, four years later, while vacationing in New Hampshire, we found ourselves at a Christian center for three weeks, where it just happened that Cay and Judy were scheduled to lead a ten-day retreat. From the announcement, we learned that they had been doing a great deal of speaking since we had seen them in 1961, and had also become involved in the healing ministry. Only a few months before, my mother had discovered that she had an advanced case of cancer and had less than six months to live. So we called her and asked her to come to New Hampshire and join us at this retreat. She came, also anxious to hear what the healing ministry was all about, and perhaps harboring the hope that God, through these two women, might do something about her cancer. She was not quite fifty years old and had a four-year-old son—my brother Brian, an unexpected but rich blessing to her and my dad.

We all learned a great deal about healing and about the work and power of God's Holy Spirit that week in New Hampshire. But most of all, we learned about the need to get our relationships with our families into the place where they were pleasing to God. Mom and I talked about a lot of hurts and misunderstandings we had while I was growing up, all the normal mother-daughter problems, plus a few that were uniquely our own.

There were four of us kids in the family. I was number two and the only girl. Boys generally get preferential treatment, and our home was no exception. I sized that situation up early in life. It was a man's world, and the only way to be at the center of attention was to beat my brothers. But the odds were insurmountable, and I began to employ more devious methods. I became Daddy's girl. That was something my brothers couldn't do, and it worked pretty well. I got the attention I wanted, but it was never enough. I became haunted by the conviction that my parents really *did* love my brothers more than me.

Through most of my later childhood and adolescence, I complained bitterly to my mother that she preferred the boys and would insist that it was true, whenever she tried to deny it. This instilled instant guilt in her and got me a lot of attention, while she repeatedly tried to prove to me it wasn't so. But the irony was that I myself had come to believe what had initially been a ploy for attention. The result was that I gradually became obsessed by a craving for acceptance and a corresponding fear of rejection.

In high school, I used my female charm as I had on my father, but on a more public scale. Whereas my older brother had been class president, I arranged to get myself appointed a drum majorette for the marching band. I got a lot more public exposure than the class president did, and my picture was all over the yearbook, too.

As I moved on through adolescence, I was reasonably confident that my charm would get me what I wanted, although inside, it wasn't long before I knew that charm wasn't enough. I continued to feel rejected, angry, and rebellious, now smoking and drinking my way into the "in" crowd. This was just the opposite from what my parents wanted for me and from what my brother was. I guess it was my way of punishing them both.

Anyway, that was my state when I graduated from high school in 1954 and promptly left home to entice the world to bow adoringly at my feet. But the world didn't go for it, and within four years I found myself wrung out, at the end of a miserable relationship, flat on my face, begging God to help me. Don't ask me why; maybe I figured He would give me what everyone else had failed to.

All by myself, sobbing uncontrollably on the floor of my apartment on a cold, wintry January night, I called out to God. "Please, *please!* Help me, God! There's got to be more in life than what I've found. I'd rather be dead than hurt like this over and over again." And indeed, the thought of suicide had been stronger in recent months and was almost a comfort in my moments of despair.

As I lay there, my despair subsided, and in its place came a new, unaccustomed peace. And from that moment, my life began to change. Though I didn't know what had happened until six months later, I had undergone, of all things, a conversion! It was an inauspicious beginning to a journey that would lead me in an entirely new direction. Christ wanted to be the *center* of my life. I had always gone to church, but now I went with a new spark of joy. I began to read the Bible whenever I could, and I knew God personally for the first time.

My parents and friends saw a difference in me. I couldn't explain it and didn't try to, but, for the first time in my life, I knew I was going in the right direction. I stopped putting such ridiculous demands on my parents' love, and I began to really love *them* and be grateful for the home and the life that they had given me. I finally became a daughter to them. Mom and I would talk for hours over a cup of tea. Many, many times we went to the retreat center in our little town, Whitinsville, for what they called "quiet days" with a beautiful Episcopalian teacher, Estelle Carver. We were blessed richly by these experiences together.

But now the news of Mom's cancer threatened to put an abrupt stop to our new relationship, and we were all hurting.

During that week in New Hampshire, she was able to talk openly about her fear of dying, her anxiety over leaving my dad with such a young son to raise, and her desire to know more of God. As she listened to Cay and Judy, she began to trust God for her own life and the life of her family. It was a tremendous relief to her to *know* that God would take care of Dad and Brian. She counseled privately with Cay and Judy, and they led her, so lovingly and gently, into facing both her life and her death in and with Jesus. Coming to grips with those facts was a deeply emotional experience for her and for me. There were times of great joy and laughing, and times of crying and weeping together.

The reality of life and death was before us continually those ten days, in a way neither of us had ever seen it. She wanted to live, but she knew that dying in Christ was even better. It was a struggle. But, in spite of the depth of emotion we were both experiencing, we found a deep, inner release from God that was unexplainable. Each day, from that time on, was a gift from God. And He extended her time with us for a whole year beyond the doctor's expectation. She died July 4, 1966. Needless to say, our reactions to Cay and Judy were no longer mixed. Bill started inviting them to our church in Bridgeport, and then to Parkminster, in Rochester, when we moved. They stayed in our home and spent evenings sitting around the living room and sharing with us about the daily reality of God, as He works in and through the people around us. It wasn't deep, theological teaching, just the truth of how Jesus works in the most mundane things of life and uses them to help us to grow. They saw God in all the little things of life, in spilled milk and broken dishes, in blossoming trees and in thunderstorms. God was a part of everything for Cay and Judy, and that's what we loved about them.

By the time of this spring luncheon in 1973, the Lord had raised up a Christian community at Rock

Harbor. A dozen families had joined with the Andersens and Sorensens, to put into practice the simple, practical truths that Cay and Judy taught.

The luncheon was an unqualified success, as Cay and Judy shared from their lives; the 250 guests were alternately moved to laughter and to solemn reflection. And it marked only the beginning of a wonderful week of learning and growth for a great many people at Parkminster, including me.

I'm a judgmental person. I didn't like it, for example, when the women serving the luncheon that day failed to serve the head table first. And I didn't like the serving dishes they had picked to use. I wanted to look good in front of Cay and Judy, and I wanted the church to look good, and so those things and more were irritating me. But as Cay and Judy began to talk about judgments and how destructive they were, I listened. And before long, tears were rolling down my cheeks through the rest of their talk. It was as if they had been aware of all my thoughts during lunch. The more they talked, the more distressed I became. It wasn't just the thoughts I had at this luncheon—I now saw that I was judging all the time.

I could not stop crying. Even when everyone else was laughing, I could hardly get a full smile on my face. I wasn't sure I was going to be able to make it through the luncheon. And I was embarrassed. I tried brushing my tears away as inconspicuously as possible—praying no one would notice. After all, I was the senior minister's wife, and I had to keep my poise in front of 250 women! Or so I thought. Bill was arranging private counseling sessions after the luncheon, for those who wanted to talk with Cay and Judy. "Do you think I could see them first?" I whispered to him. I felt like I had to get my judgments out to Cay and Judy quickly, before I could be of any use to Bill or the church or my family. So I became the first in line for private counseling in the chapel.

The moment I walked in and saw them, I burst out crying. "I'm a mess and I really need help!" "Here, Carol," Judy said, smiling and handing me a Kleenex. "What seems to be going on in you?"

I expected a two-hour counseling session, but in less than ten minutes it was over. "Let God continue to convict you of your judgments and show you more of your wrong attitudes at church and at home. Stop trying to relieve the pressure you're under—let it work for you." I assured them I would take their advice, but underneath I think I was miffed that they took so little time with me. They didn't seem the least bit concerned. I felt overwhelmed and shocked at what I had just learned about myself. The minister's wife of this large Presbyterian church in Rochester was full of judgments towards dozens of people in the church. What a lousy Christian I was! Why weren't they more surprised?

The mission continued. Cay and Judy talked about how difficult it was for Christians to be wrong. "Christians don't seem to understand that Christ is the only righteous one," Judy said. "When you see that you are wrong, then you see how much you need Jesus. It is your wrongness that entitles you to a Savior." I had never seen that before. After I had committed my life to God, I thought I could no longer be really wrong about anything. A good Christian was supposed to do everything right, so I kept my ugly thoughts hidden, as if they weren't even there. But invariably, the thought—or a worse one—would come back. I was living in a pretend world.

Cay and Judy told us that Jesus died for our wrongness. We did not have to work, work, work at being right, but instead we had to flee to Jesus in our wrongness. I didn't know exactly what that meant, but I wanted to find out. I was seeing my need for Jesus Christ as I had not seen it before. When I was converted fourteen years before, I knew that I needed Christ to change my life and save me from some pretty ugly sins. But I didn't realize, until this mission, how much I needed Him every day. Left to myself, I was jealous, critical, and judgmental of everyone around me. Oh, I seldom expressed these thoughts directly, but they consumed a great deal of my time, and I knew it. And so did God.

The mission began at the noon luncheon on Monday and lasted until Thursday afternoon. Every minute was busy. Cay and Judy taught morning and evening sessions and counseled individuals each afternoon. I wanted to ask a million questions and get all kinds of personal attention, but I remembered their counsel. "Let it work for you, Carol—don't take God's pressure off yourself. "And I had felt progressively lighter and freer as the week went on. I felt God's hand on me, convicting me and then forgiving me. It was amazing! It had been a long time since I had felt the presence of God so continually in my life—all day long!

Just before they were about to leave, I had another opportunity to talk with them. "I've seen so much about myself during this week, but I don't know how to begin to change. I see very clearly what a critical, judgmental person I am. And I've begun to see how much I have hurt the people around me with this attitude. But what do I do about it?" "It takes time to overcome the attitudes of judgment that you have indulged in for years. But it can be done," Cay smiled. "Why don't you submit yourself to a discipline for a specific period of time. That's what we find works at the Community." "What do you mean? What kind of discipline?" "A self-imposed discipline not to say a critical word about anything for a certain period of time," she answered. "Sure, I'll do that, but whom would I submit to?" "How about Bill?" Judy asked. "I'd be delighted!" he responded abruptly. "Frankly, I'm sick and tired of listening to all of her judgments. I'm constantly defeated by her critical attitude towards me and the children."

I winced. It was one thing for me to admit my problem; it was another to have Bill confirm it so bluntly. I pulled back, and they noticed. I hated to think anyone, including Bill, was aware of my sin. I thought I had concealed it. I didn't speak, but the hurt was written all over my face. My ugliness had not been hidden at all, and I was embarrassed by Bill's quick comments. My pretend world was crumbling fast. "Don't be so hurt by Bill's honesty," Judy said. "You need to see that sin does affect those around you. It should make you want to change even more."

I knew she was right, but I was having a difficult time coming up over the feelings I was having. And now I was getting really angry at Bill for exposing me like that. And Judy's next suggestion only made it worse. "I think you should be under a discipline not to say a critical word to Bill for three months. And he should help you keep this discipline." *Three months! Three whole months without saying one critical thing? I'll never make it!*" "By God's grace, you can, Carol, if you really want to," Cay said gently. "Pray about it and see if that's not what God would have you do. Strong habit patterns need radical steps to overcome the hold they have on our lives, because they pull us away from God."

She spoke with such compassion—like she knew exactly how difficult it would be. But she also spoke with confidence and faith that God would help it all to happen a lot more easily than I could imagine at that moment. "Stick with it, and it will begin a new work in your life," Judy said, getting into the car. And before we knew it they were on their way back to Cape Cod, looking almost as refreshed and renewed as they had when they had arrived.

I was wiped out. I felt like I had been working ten hours a day since Monday, and there was not an ounce of strength left in me. How could I possibly begin a discipline like the one they had suggested? That would take more fight than I had in me.

I wanted to just forget their suggestion, but Bill didn't let me.

I had all kinds of reasons why I couldn't possibly go on such a discipline. "God will give you the strength you need," Bill said confidently. "I really believe He has spoken through Cay and Judy, and now you must act on what you've heard."

❧

The first two weeks on the discipline were awful. It seemed like my whole life had been one monstrous judgment. I could hardly speak a sentence that didn't begin, "I don't like the . . ." or, "Why didn't you . . ." or, "Your tie doesn't. . . ." My hand was over my mouth most of the time. "I'm sorry, Bill," seemed to be the only thing I could say for days. It was hard, but I was coming to see myself as I never had before. And I was grieved at what I saw. I had been tearing down my relationship with Bill and the children. And

I asked God to forgive and change me—using this period of three months to start the change process.

The things that upset me—the top being left off the toothpaste, the newspaper beside the bed in the morning, the phone calls made just before dinner was served— were so trivial. But I used to badger my family to death with my complaints. I think Bill and the kids had become almost deaf to me, so that, if I had ever had anything important to say, they probably couldn't have heard me. For three months I had to look for things to be grateful for, instead of poisoning the air with criticisms, morning, noon, and night. And this was especially true at meal times, when I customarily let each member of the family know just where he or she was failing around the house. "Tim, the wastebaskets didn't get emptied again. You are so lazy and forgetful." "Betsy, your room was a mess. When are you going to learn how to be neat?" "Peter, if I find the Legos out of their box again, I'll get rid of them and spank you." "The dog's dishes weren't washed." "There are toys out in the yard that need to be put away." On and on the litany of complaint went, meal after meal.

Yes, the children did need to hear those things every day, in order to be taught responsibility, but my attitude was terrible. There was absolutely nothing any of them could do to satisfy me. I wasn't telling them those things to help them at all; instead of constructive criticism, it was destructive.

So, for this period of time, Bill took the full responsibility to keep the children in tow with their various chores around the house. I needed Bill's help so much. And how I needed God! I was forced to pray all day, not on my knees with my eyes closed and hands folded, but just continuously talking to Him. "God, help me with what I saw this morning. And give me a grateful heart tonight at dinner." I was beginning to understand how God could be an active part of all the events of our home, no matter how small and mundane they seemed. And it was different for me to need God and Bill so much.

I had disciplined myself many times before in my life—for a period of time—and with some sort of goal in mind. But never had I needed or desired the moment-by-moment help of anyone else, including God.

In Weight Watchers, the lecturer would say, "Before you know it, your tastes will change. You won't want to eat those foods you now love so much." To me, that meant that someday I would not have to even bother to resist; my desires would be gone, and it would all just happen without any more effort on my part. But that day never came for me. I still loved apple pie and chocolate ice cream as much as ever. The self-imposed discipline helped me to achieve my goal weight, but it didn't change my desires at all. And, whenever I cheated on my diet or gained any weight, I would just stay away from the meetings. That way, I didn't have to face my failure.

God had to be a part of any change that was going to happen in my life, if it was going to last. And for my own good, someone close to me had to be involved with imposing that discipline on me—in this case, Bill. It put me in a very safe position of not being able to do it alone.

My feeling about discipline had been that it was a form of punishment and was used only to correct outward behavior. But now I saw the possibility of it being used by God to work a change deep inside of me. In fact, not only did I see that possibility, I felt it happening to me. At the beginning of the three months, I felt like I was tied up with a thick rope, not able to move without pain. That changed. Instead of my feeling bound, the opposite was happening, and I was feeling free: free from my damnable judgments and critical attitude toward my husband and children. And, funny thing, I was literally falling in love anew with my family.

THREE

The Sand of Cape Cod

Brrrrinng . . . Brrrrinng. . . . "I'm coming, just a minute!" I yelled up from the family room at the telephone ringing itself off the wall in the kitchen. Why did that phone always have to ring just when I was in the middle of loading the washer? Knowing how easily I could get involved on the phone, I shoved the load in quickly and ran upstairs. "Hello?" I answered breathlessly. "Carol, sorry to bother you"—the phone had rung a good ten times before I had answered. "I—I really need help." The voice was shaky and scared. I tried to attach a face to it. The woman was crying and talking at the same time, and was desperately trying to control the crying. "School has been out only two weeks, and I can't bear to think about the whole summer. . . . I'll never make it!" And now she was sobbing in between her words. "Not only are the children home all day, but of course Bob is, too."

I had the face now; it was Lois, a very bright but insecure mother who had recently joined the church. Her husband, Bob, taught school in the city, and they had two young active children. I had had lunch with her not too long ago at another parishioner's home.

I didn't know Lois well, but that day at lunch I had begun to be concerned for her. She was extremely uptight about a project she had undertaken at her daughter Jenny's elementary school. Ruth and I had suggested that she make an appointment with Bill for some counseling. The last I heard, she had stopped working on the project, and her uptightness had lifted noticeably. But that was hardly the case today. "I just can't stand the confusion around here! Bob just left with the children for the day. I suppose he hopes that will help me, but I know it will be the same when he gets home." She started crying again. "It seemed like I just got on my feet from that whole mess at Jenny's school, and now the summer vacation is pulling me down. It's just one thing after another."

There was a long pause. "I actually considered running away—just for a few days. I have a good bike and a pup tent, and I could find a secluded place alone somewhere and try to get my head together." (I really felt like laughing, as I pictured her riding through the middle of town on her bike with a pup tent, but I knew she was serious, and that this was not the time to laugh.) "The next thing I thought about doing was going to the liquor store and buying a bottle of something and getting drunk." (I was pretty sure she didn't drink, so this, too, made me want to laugh.) "But," she went on, "I knew that when I sobered up, I still would have to face my family and myself."

Another long pause. I slipped into a comfortable chair in the living room, realizing this was going to be a long telephone call. Thank God for ten-foot-long telephone cords! "My third choice was to call you for help. Can you, will you, help me?" "Of course, Lois," I said, "I'm not sure how, but I will if I can." And as she went on, sounding somewhat relieved, I suddenly became aware of what I was getting into. Why didn't she call Bill? He's the trained counselor, not me! I tried to pray as she talked, but my own questions kept inter-rupting my prayers. *I hope she's not suicidal. Lord, what in the world can I do for her?*

She just went on expressing the hopeless state of confusion she felt. "Is there any way out?" she finally asked with a desperate edge to her voice.

Now the pause was on my end of the telephone line; I had no idea what to say to her. The words that finally came out floored me. "Lois, I think I'm supposed to come over today, but not to talk to you. And I think I'm supposed to bring someone with me. And the three of us are supposed to clean your house." *What in the world had I said?* I had never been in Lois's house and had no idea whether it needed cleaning. And further-more, what business was it of mine whether or not it did need cleaning? The thought had just popped into my head and out of my mouth.

She burst out laughing. And I felt like a jerk. "You're going to come over and help me clean my house? What makes you think I need help around the house?"

I didn't even attempt to answer that. "Lois, that's what I think I'm supposed to do to help you," I said, getting a little irritated. "Do you want my help or not?"

She laughed some more. Again, I felt stupid for even offering to do such a thing, and I wished now I could just hang up the phone. "Sure, I'd love to have you come over and clean for me." By this time, I didn't want to go, but I still had the feeling that that was what God wanted. "Okay, I'll be over as soon as I can." I stood there, staring at the phone, half wishing that I had never answered it. *Now what was I going to do? God, help me.* I could think of a dozen things I needed to do around my own house. I had a choice at that moment, standing there, between going to Lois's and forgetting the whole thing. Everything in me wanted to call her back and tell her to go see Bill and get the real help she needed. But when I picked up the phone, I dialed Helene, my reliable babysitter, instead. I explained that I needed her help for a special project and wondered if she would be willing. "Sure, Mrs. Showalter, I wasn't busy at all—I'd be glad to help." Boy, was I grateful. There was no way I wanted to go alone to a strange house and clean with an emotional woman I hardly knew.

So, off we went. More questions harassed me on the drive over. What if her husband comes back? Will he be angry, finding me in their house, cleaning? What if she is too upset to clean? Maybe I've insulted her with my offer? How could I have been so presumptuous!

We pulled into her driveway, or at least what I hoped was her driveway. "Helene, would you look in my pocketbook and see if I jotted down the house number?" She was rustling through some papers when I saw Lois at the front door. "Never mind, there's Lois now."

Lois was trying to greet us with a smile, but it was a hurt, scared smile. "Come on in. The house is a mess, and I'm a mess, too. But you already know that, or you wouldn't be here," she said with a nervous laugh. For a moment the three of us just stood there in the darkened living room, tense and uncomfortable.

The draperies were closed, making the house appear very dark and dreary. There were toys scattered around the floor, but certainly nothing unusually out of order. Beyond the living room, I could see a dining area and the kitchen. Although it was nearly eleven o'clock, the breakfast dishes were waiting to be loaded into the dishwasher, and the cereal boxes were still out on the table. What were we supposed to do now?

There didn't seem to be a nice, smooth way to get into this, so I just jumped in. "Helene, why don't you go out to the kitchen and start cleaning up the counters and doing the dishes."

"Sure," she answered, and off she went. I had explained to her in the car, as best I could, what I thought we would be doing, and she thought it was a great idea to help someone out like this. Her enthusiasm helped me, since I had come to think that it was not such a good idea! "Lois, if you'll get the vacuum out and some dust cloths and furniture polish, I'll start in right here," I said, pointing to the living room area. "How about laundry? Are you all caught up?" I asked.

Another outburst of laughter. It seemed her laughing was almost as spontaneous as her crying. "Caught up? There are at least three loads downstairs to wash and several more to fold and put away." "Okay, why don't you make that your project for a few hours."

I noticed a large stereo console at the other end of the living room, and the thought came to me to suggest we listen to some good Christian music, so I did. Lois was delighted. I found out she loved music and, in fact, wanted to take piano lessons as soon as she could find time. Before going off to the laundry room, she put on a record of favorite hymns.

The first thing I did was to pull back the draperies. Then I opened the front door and a couple of windows to let in the warm July air. The darkness lifted immediately, and the music encouraged us in our tasks.

I had to leave at noon, but Helene volunteered to carry on after lunch, if I would come back for her later in the afternoon.

When I returned, about three o'clock, Bob and the children were home, and they were all smiles. Lois's mood was totally different. "I feel so much better!" she called out to me in the driveway, loudly enough for the neighbors to hear, I feared. "I don't know how on earth cleaning the house could make such a difference—it usually works just the opposite way on me and makes me more depressed," she said, walking over towards me. "I know it helped me to have you and Helene here. Thanks a million." "It did seem like a pretty strange answer to your upset and tears," I laughed, "but it worked, and we can thank God for that."

Helene talked all the way home about what fun she had working with Lois. "And guess what?" she exclaimed. "She wants me to come back two or three mornings for the next few weeks, and she'll pay me! Which is great, because I need to save some money for the church's senior high retreat in September."

I shook my head in wonder at how it had all worked out. Bill was astounded when I told him about it that evening. "Honey," he chuckled, "you've just broken every rule in counseling. Here I am, about to get my doctorate in the subject, and never have I heard or read anywhere that the answer to a woman's depression is for the counselor to run over and clean her house." He laughed. "And since when do ministers' wives offer cleaning services as part of their jobs?" And now we both laughed. "I don't know much about counseling, but you have to admit it worked. And if housecleaning did the trick, maybe it *should* be in one of your text books!"

We laughed some more, but inside we both felt very grateful to God. Bill had counseled Lois in the past, and he felt it was a real miracle that her depression had lifted so quickly.

Several weeks later, Lois called again early one morning. She wasn't the same woman. "Oh, I still have all those problems I mentioned to you that day on the phone, but I feel one hundred percent better about them all. I know God is going to see me through. I don't feel desperate or hopeless any more." And there was hope in her voice, and trust—so different from that time a few weeks earlier. We decided to get together and sit down and work out a daily plan for her housework and her needs with the children. It was clear to both of us that when things were confused around the house, it affected her emotionally. As long as Bob and the children were at school, a certain schedule was imposed in their household. But when school was out, that schedule evaporated. So we both agreed she needed her own schedule, and she asked me to help her make one.

Naturally, a summer schedule would be different from one for school days. The children could stay up a little later, and Bob and she could sleep in a little in the mornings. But lunchtime was set at quarter past twelve, instead of everyone just eating when they got hungry. It had turned out in the past that with no time set for lunch, it ran from 11:30, when little Andy felt hungry, to 1:15, when Bob got around to eating, thus dragging it out far too long for Lois. We also decided on specific times for the two other meals, and then we loosely divided the day into housework chores in the morning and kids' activities and shopping in the afternoon.

Lois was genuinely excited about the prospect of running the house in the summer with some sort of organization. And Bob, too, was well pleased, responding to it enthusiastically and supporting Lois in implementing it right away.

As they left church the following Sunday, Bob waited outside of the door for a few minutes to speak to us. "Things are so different around our house these past few weeks, you wouldn't believe it! And we are all feeling a lot better. I really appreciate all you've done." His eyes filled, as he put his hand out to shake hands with Bill. My eyes filled, too, and I reached out and gave him a big hug.

✍

"Just think, Dad, only eight more days, and then no more telephone calls for a whole month!" Those were the words of our son, Tim, as August approached. Tomorrow it would be "just think, Dad, only seven more days. . . ." August—Bill's vacation month—was just around the corner, and soon we'd be off to Cape Cod, our favorite spot.

Our first Cape Cod vacation had been in the early 1960s, when the grandfather of a girl in our church in Bridgeport gave us the keys to his cottage for a month. We loved it and had a glorious time, but never felt we could afford to go back. Instead, we tried various attempts at vacationing, none of which was very acceptable: Christian camps, where the cost was low and the spiritual activity high; and then "visit the family," which was never very relaxing. So we kept searching, not quite satisfied with our vacations, hoping someday to find the perfect spot. It was important to get away from the phone and appointments and just relax, but at the same time we also knew that we needed some spiritual intake during that month, or the busy fall schedule would overwhelm us.

Then it had happened. In addition to Rock Harbor Manor, the guesthouse that Bill and Cay Andersen owned in Orleans on Cape Cod, they had a small cottage that they rented out during the summer. It sounded just like what we were looking for—two bedrooms, a kitchen, a bath, and a front room, snuggled in a quiet grove of locust trees behind the guesthouse, only a five-minute walk to the beach. We had rented it, sight unseen, for the month of August 1966. Our family loved it. And there was lots of Christian fellowship to be had. Twice a week, on Monday and Thursday evenings, in the living room of the guesthouse, there was a time of sharing and teaching, open to anyone who wanted to come. There we met people from all over New England as well as from the Cape—vacationers who, like us, wanted more than just a vacation.

We looked forward to those informal gatherings in such gracious surroundings. Cay and Judy would sit on a sofa, and I had never seen two people who could share as easily as they. Their words blended together as if only one person were speaking. One would pause and the other would begin, and the unbroken continuity of their thoughts was amazing. And not only did their words blend beautifully, and their personalities, but Cay's blond hair and light complexion complemented Judy's dark hair and eyes. Even the colors in their dresses were compatible, never drawing attention to themselves, but each deferring to the other. It was a joy and privilege to sit and listen and watch these two women whom God had obviously set apart for a special call in life.

Sometimes there would be as many as forty people sitting in the spacious living room, including six or seven ministers and their wives. As Cay and Judy shared, Bill from time to time would leaf through his Bible for the pertinent Scripture reference, but I just sat, captivated by the life of Christ I saw and sensed coming through them. And when the meeting was over, no one wanted to leave. It was fun just standing around, talking to one another and getting acquainted.

After a while, many of us regulars began to get together at other times during the week. An Episcopal priest, Father Arthur Lane, of St. Paul's in Darien, Connecticut, had a beautiful waterfront cottage in Harwichport, to which he and his wife would invite us for a day of picnicking and swimming. For us, Monday and Thursday nights soon became times to meet with friends as well as to learn more about the down-to-earth practicalities of daily living in Christ.

We returned to that cottage at Rock Harbor the next summer, and in fact for the next four summers. Change, however, was inevitable around the quiet guesthouse and cottage. The Christian community that was rapidly growing up there became officially incorporated on June 19, 1970.

I'll never forget what happened the first Sunday morning we were there that summer. Bill had decided to sleep out on the porch in a sleeping bag to fully enjoy the warm summer evening. About eight-thirty in the morning, half awake, I heard the strangest thumping around on the porch. I jumped up and could hardly believe my eyes! Bill was trying to make his way into the living room—still in the sleeping bag! He was standing upright and holding it up, or trying to hold it up, with one hand, while giving me some kind of frantic signal with the other. His finger was up over his lips and then pointed outside.

"There's church going on out there in the locust grove, he whispered. "Art has his surplice on and is conducting a communion service."

I looked out the living room window, my eyes widening. Sure enough, there was Father Lane, standing behind a small table that was serving as an altar. He had a long white robe on and was reading from the prayer book. The wind was lifting the ends of the white cloth that covered the table, and the candles were flickering. There were four neat rows of folding chairs that had not been there when we went to bed. And standing in front of them were some guests and the thirty or so people who had become a part of the Community of Jesus. They were more than just a group of people buying houses in the area—they were obviously already a family, sharing their faith in God.

Bill and I had recently talked about the changes we saw happening around the little cottage. The locust grove seemed to have become a center of activity almost daily, with volleyball games and croquet and a mid-afternoon coffee hour. We had mixed emotions— happiness for these families who seemed to have a very special relationship with one another—but sadness too, that we were losing our quiet, secluded hideaway.

I think we both knew, although neither of us said anything, that when we turned in our key that Labor Day, we would not be renting the cottage again. There was sadness deep inside me when, as we started up the old Dodge, the kids called out, "Goodbye, cottage, until next year." I wondered where we would be next August.

೭ಿ

Where we would be, it turned out, was as far in the opposite direction as possible. The following summer, 1971, we loaded the new family station wagon to the gunwales and headed west. Horses, mountains, camping—we spent most of our month immersed in a completely different kind of vacation. And it was a good trip, but though we seldom mentioned it, we found ourselves missing the fellowship at the Community. It seemed that we had a lot more than just the sand in our shoes from the Cape; we had a deep love in our heart for our summer friends. It seemed that the Cape had become far more special to us than we had realized.

After nearly three weeks of the West we found ourselves on our way home, about ten days sooner than we planned. And coincidentally, we found that we had just enough time left in our vacation month to take a fast trip to the Cape. Our station wagon went right by the Rochester exits and on towards the Massachusetts Turnpike. There were no complaints from the family, and although there were few words spoken between Bill and me, there was a mutual agreement that we were now headed in the right direction.

As we drove over the Sagamore Bridge onto the Cape, we both sensed a distinct feeling of coming home. I think it was then that we finally accepted what our hearts had known for some time—that Cape Cod had become far more than a vacation spot to us. The next summer we rented a cottage a few minutes from the Community, and just before we went back to Rochester we made a major commitment. We bought a piece of land, with the dream of building a cottage of our own as soon as possible.

FOUR

3D

August 1973 was unusually warm, and I was delighted to be able to have dinner out on the patio of our little rented cottage. The sun was setting, the mosquitoes were bearable, and the air was delightful. Hot plates, cut celery, plenty of ice in the iced tea—everything was ready, and Peter and Edith, friends of ours, were due in a few minutes. My last-minute checklist continued— the bread cups were out of the oven, crisp and browned perfectly, and would soon be filled with a shrimp-cheese Newburg. The garden asparagus was washed and ready for cooking. The smell of fresh-baked blueberry buckle filled the cottage with a most inviting aroma.

I stopped for a moment and listened to the evening. Cape Cod was so inundated with visitors that you could almost hear the hum of activity. In two weeks, the day after Labor Day, the Cape would be silent and peaceful, but right now, the tourist season was at its peak. I took a last look at the table and went to get out of my apron. They would be coming any minute. Peter and Edith were leaving shortly, to get away on a canoe trip to Maine with a group from their church, and we wanted to touch base with them before they left.

The doorbell rang around seven, and that was the last time I looked at the clock. Once again, time seemed to fly by, and the dinner by candlelight outside tasted good. Before I knew it, it was time for dessert. I brought out the warm blueberry buckle, piled high with whipped cream and sprinkled with fresh blueberries. Serving the others and then putting an ample portion down at my own place, I remarked lightly, "Oh well, I'll start my diet again tomorrow."

Edith picked up on that comment and said, "Do you remember that group I told you about that met during February and March at our church?"

I thought for a moment. "I do remember something about a group that you started, to help people with different problems, including weight. Is that the one you mean?" "That's the one," she said. "You know, it turned out to be a real blessing for a lot of people, including me."

It was quite a story to hear. She shared how a group of people had sat around a big maple table at the home of some close friends. Peter and Edith were frustrated with the needs of the people in their church. They seemed to have so many practical problems, like finances and housework and dieting and drinking, and even nail biting! Peter knew how to preach and his faith was exuberant, but getting faith down to the practical, nitty-gritty problems facing these Cape Cod families wasn't working.

After listening to all the different problems of the church people, Cay Andersen smiled and said, "Well, it sounds to me like all the problems you have been talking about come down to diet, discipline, and discipleship—3 big D's!" She laughed and her eyes twinkled with the simple answer God had given her to a very complex problem.

Everyone around the table responded enthusiastically, and the decision was made to start a support-group program that would be Christ-centered. It would deal with dieting, drinking, finances, and any other areas that would respond to self-discipline.

Now Peter picked up the narrative, continuing with a grin. "God took charge from there on," he explained. "I announced the meeting the next Sunday and made it pretty clear that certain unnamed members had better seriously consider this group for the help they needed." He chuckled. "Before we knew it, more than fifty people were ready for a six-week program."

Peter and Edith felt that they were not supposed to lead the group themselves, so they turned to the Community of Jesus, asking for some leadership. Cay and Judy encouraged two ministers' wives to go over to Peter and Edith's church—Jane, who had recently shed more than fifty pounds herself, and Lenny, who had studied nutrition. "It went so well," said Edith, "that at the end of the six weeks we had agreed upon, Lenny and Jane offered to continue a group at the Community for any who were interested in going on. From all reports, we heard everyone was very happy with the results. I lost my ten pounds in the six weeks, so I was more than satisfied." She paused, and then remembered something. "Oh! Guess what we named the group?" Edith laughed. "3D—for Diet, Discipline and Discipleship."

For no reason, just then into my mind popped the image of that red "smile" face in the East Hall at church. Now what did that have to do with—could *this* be God's answer?

Suddenly I had a million questions to ask. But it was late, and it would have been wrong to hold our guests any longer. As they were leaving, I said, "Edith, when we get back to Rochester, and you get back from Maine, I'd like to give you a call to get some more details about the 3D thing." That was all that was said, but that night I could not get to sleep. The little that Peter and Edith had shared had started an avalanche of thoughts in my head. It was like being given just one lick of a mocha almond ice-cream cone—I wanted much more!

For the remainder of our vacation, I could hardly get my mind off 3D. Bill and I were sitting on the beach one afternoon, watching the children swim, when for the umpteenth time, I started wondering who back home might be interested in such a group. And the list of questions I wanted to ask Edith grew longer and longer. But Edith was off in Maine canoeing, so I pestered Bill instead. "Bill?" "Mm?" he said, absorbed in *Time* magazine. "Do you think Dorcas might be interested, hon?" "Interested in what?" he murmured, not looking up. "Interested in a 3D group back at church." "Maybe." "I bet Margaret and Dee would be, because of their weight problem, don't you?" "Well," he replied, throwing me a quick glance, "I suppose you won't know till you get home and ask them, right?" And he turned back to *Time*.

I knew all he wanted was to read in peace, but it didn't seem fair that he should be so peaceful when I was anything but. "Hon, Edith said she was able to lose ten pounds during the six weeks. . . . I haven't lost ten pounds in the last year, trying by myself."

No answer, not even a grunt. "I'll bet Norma would love to be involved in a Christian weight group—and MaryJane is anxious to take off the weight she gained since Kirk was born. That's already five others besides me for a group, and I'll bet Lois would join, too."

No answer—then "Mmf" as I poked him in the side. "Hey, take it easy!" he chuckled, grabbing my wrist. "Sounds to me like that group has already started, but you haven't talked to one person yet. What's more, there's no way you can talk to anyone until we get back to Rochester. So why don't you put this whole 3D thing out of your mind and enjoy the last of our vacation. Remember, it will be a whole year before we can get back here." And he put the magazine over his eyes and settled himself for a snooze.

Bill was right, of course. It was typical of me to get so wrapped up in something that I forgot everything else. I needed to be thinking about my family and our vacation and not some new program. There would be lots of time for that after Labor Day.

So I did the best I could. I stopped talking about it—but it was more than I could do to stop thinking about it.

Before we knew it, Labor Day had arrived. And that meant that we would leave, at five the next morning, for our long journey home. What a blessing that one extra day after the holidays was! The traveling was much easier with most of the vacationers already off the Cape and back home.

We tucked boxes and bags into every conceivable corner of the station wagon, and strapped the suitcases onto the luggage rack on the roof. We locked the cottage door, and off we went. It was one of those perfect driving days—sunny, but breezy too, with fluffy white clouds scudding across the sky. As soon as we passed the Albany exits on the thruway, we began to get anxious for the sight and sound of Rochester. For some reason, Albany and east seemed to be the Cape Cod side of the trip, and everything west of Albany meant we were nearing home. It was funny how certain places had become landmarks on our many trips to and from Cape Cod—the bridge to the mainland, our breakfast stop at the Friendly's in Auburn, the two Albany exits, the cheap gas and ice cream stop in Herkimer, and then Rochester.

The children couldn't wait to call their friends the minute we got in the door, and Bill couldn't wait to get his mail from the office. I couldn't wait to get the suitcases emptied and get settled in our own rooms and know we'd be sleeping in our very own beds. And once all the baths and shampoos were over, and the new school clothes were laid out on the beds, and prayers said on that Tuesday night, we knew vacation was far behind us.

❧

The buzz around Parkminster was always fantastic in September. It was exhilarating to go over and watch all the activity—the preschool teachers and aides scrubbing and cleaning, the Sunday school staff getting the nursery and the other classrooms ready, and various people painting and cleaning around the church. Choir rehearsals and youth groups would be starting the first Wednesday in September, and the leaders were busy getting music and materials ready. The moment the kids were off to school Wednesday morning, I put on my jacket and took the familiar walk across the yard to the church.

I recognized Jean's car in the parking lot. Jean was the program chairman for the women's association and one of the most active women in our church; she would be the perfect one to try out 3D on!

And just then, as if on cue, she came hurrying out. "Hi, Carol, welcome home!" she said, pausing on her way to her car. "Hope you had a good, restful vacation on Cape Cod." "We did! We enjoyed every minute, as usual."

I could see she was in a hurry, but I didn't want to let her go until I at least mentioned 3D. "Jean, I learned about the most exciting group that met at a church on Cape Cod last winter and at the Community of Jesus. It really sounds like just what we need around—" "I'd love to hear about it," she said, opening the door of her car. "Maybe we can get together after the fall luncheon."

After the fall luncheon! My heart sank. That meant October! "I guess I thought it was something we could maybe start soon, like next week . . . and I—"

"Oh, Carol," she said, trying to say it kindly, but revealing the pressure she was under, "there's no way I can even think about another program until next spring! And I still have to find committee chairmen for several openings that have come up over the summer months."

From my own term as program chairman, I should have appreciated all the pressure she was under, but I didn't appreciate anything but 3D. "It's called a diet, discipline and discipleship group," I went on hurriedly, "and, in a sense, it is a Christ-oriented counterpart of Weight Watchers. The Bible is used, and prayer is a basic tool to help women get more disciplined in—" "Carol, please forgive me, but I've got to run. I'm late for a luncheon committee meeting. It's great to have you back again." And she waved, as she got in her car and closed the door.

Standing there and watching her back out and pull away, I waved, but inside I felt like crying. I tried to tell myself how busy she was, and how unfair it had been of me to grab her and spring 3D on her. But I was also thinking that she had such a good figure and no problem or any lack of self-discipline, so of course she wouldn't be interested.

I tried also to remind myself, walking into the church, that if this were indeed God's answer, it would somehow all work out. But not even the smell of fresh paint or the happy bustle of activity could lift my spirits. I started wandering toward the preschool activity. Then, I heard my name called. "Carol? Well, Carol! Welcome home!" It was Dorcas, the wife of our assistant minister. "I saw you talking to Jean outside. Did she tell you that they've sold over a hundred tickets already for the luncheon, and it's still three weeks away?" "Say, that's great!" I said feebly, "She certainly is busy." I realized with chagrin that I had never even asked Jean about how the luncheon was coming.

"For a supposedly quiet month," Dorcas went on, "August has been absolutely incredible around here. I hope it was quieter for you all at the Cape." "We did see Peter and Edith a few times and had a great time visiting the Community of Jesus. There are more than eighty resident members there now, and all keeping busy from the look of things. They've got a new chapel—you wouldn't recognize the place. But I guess the most exciting thing I heard was about a new support group." "Oh, you mean their Upper Room Fellowship?" "No," I said, happy that I could surprise her, "a group called 3D—diet, discipline and discipleship." "Ugh, diet! Don't even mention that word to me—please! I joined Weight Watchers and quit again, just in the month you've been away." She laughed. "I think I'm going to get a pin for being the person who has joined and quit the most in one year." I managed a weak smile. It was plain to see she was not the least bit interested in any diet group—Christian or otherwise. I didn't say any more, but inside I had the feeling that walls were caving in. I felt so down and rejected by both Jean's and Dorcas's reaction. . . . Had I really heard God?

FIVE

THE FAT, THE SLEEPY, AND THE SLOPPY

September began to slip away, day by day. I didn't bring up the subject of 3D again to anyone. In my hurt and rejection I decided that dieting and discipline were just not important enough to hassle about. And little by little the bathroom scale went up, as I enjoyed French fries, Toll House cookies, and ice cream cones whenever I could sneak them in. I was eating and enjoying it, and to heck with every thought of dieting!

One night after dinner, I suggested the whole family go out for dessert. Bill raised his eyebrows and said, "Hey, how come all these desserts and treats lately? I thought you were all gung-ho on this diet thing after we got home from the Cape." He paused. "Whatever happened to that 3D idea?" "No one was interested," I muttered, getting up from the table to clear the dishes and hopefully end the discussion. "What do you mean, no interest? You had enough excitement and interest on Cape Cod for ten people. And, when you get something in your head, you take off and get it together. Now come back here and sit down, and let's get to the bottom of this. What's the real problem?"

I told him how I felt, and that Jean was right; we already did have so much going on at church—"and there really isn't any time to start a new program around here. Maybe next year—" "Carol," Bill cut me off, "I think you're being vindictive about the whole 3D thing because Jean and Dorcas didn't buy your idea immediately. You've never really sought God's will on this. All you've done is withdraw."

He was right. I had not worked through the thing at all, just shelved the whole idea. And soothed my hurt by doing just the absolute opposite of dieting—eating anything and everything I wanted. "It seems to me," he continued, "that you named six or seven others who you were sure would be interested. So why don't you talk to them and a few others about it?" And most important, we both agreed to pray seriously about it. If the idea was from God, Bill concluded, He would surely let us know soon.

✌

"Anyone home?" called a voice outside our side door. "Sure," I called out, "come on in.

In walked Lois, bright, cheerful and excited. "I just wanted to stop by and tell you how well the summer went!" She was beaming. "It's been the best summer we've ever had! That schedule you worked out with me in July was a gift from God to me and my family."

She waited for me to respond. For a minute I couldn't remember what she was talking about, and then it dawned on me. "Oh, I'd almost forgotten about that. But I'll never forget that fun day we had cleaning!"

I was frankly amazed at her excitement and freedom. She really was different. We sat and talked and then looked over her schedule. And it looked great—beautifully organized. "Carol, I wonder . . . well, would you mind if I checked in with you on a regular basis, just to keep things going in the right direction?"

"Sure, as long as you don't expect me to come and clean every week," I laughed. It was a joy seeing Lois so free—so absolutely different from that encounter in July.

The next day, I had another surprise visitor. "Your husband felt I ought to come over and tell you what I just told him," Norma started. "As you know, I've lost a great deal of weight since the beginning of the year, and now I've even started lecturing in the Diet Workshop group I belong to." "I didn't know that you were lecturing, Norma; that's great!" "Well, I'm not sure it's so great. The reason I was able to lose the weight had more to do with my new faith in God than the diet program itself; and that really makes it hard, because I have to sell a diet program—and not talk about God at all."

I just shook my head. "Bill tells me you are thinking about starting a diet group based on Christian principles," she continued. "I think it sounds tremendous! I'd love to be a part of it, if possible."

I must have had a surprised look on my face. "Thanks, Norma. I did think about that very seriously and then kind of dropped the idea. But it's beginning to seem more possible now."

We talked awhile, and I assured her I would get in touch with her when the plans became more concrete.

And in a few hours, I had a third unexpected visitor. Ruth walked in, nervously stopping at the top step before coming in the kitchen. "I'm sorry to just drop in this way, but Bill said he thought it would be good if I came over and talked to you. . . ." Then she burst out crying. Ruth was an attractive woman with light brown hair and soft facial features. As she spoke, her voice was almost mousy-quiet and squeaky—and because of the tears, I could hardly understand her.

"Come in the living room, Ruth, and sit down," I said, putting my arm around her shoulder. Our living room had two love seats; she sat on one, and I sat opposite her on the other. For a few minutes she cried, and I sat there, praying silently. Her crying was coming from so deep inside, it made me hurt. I felt helpless sitting there, but I knew it was good for her just to cry, no matter how uncomfortable we both were. "I find it really hard to talk to anyone, Carol . . . especially about my personal life. I'm a person who doesn't let people get too close to me, and I don't get too close to them." Her voice was shaky and the crying continued in between pauses. "All I want to do lately is sleep, sleep, sleep. The minute Dan leaves for work and the children go to school, I go back to bed and sleep half the morning away. Then, believe it or not, I go back to bed after lunch and sleep half the afternoon. I just don't want to be with anyone or do anything." She started crying hard again. "The minute people begin to get close to me, I pull away." "What can I do to help, Ruth?" I asked. "I don't know. . . . I don't know if anyone can help me. I'm running from my responsibilities, and I'm running from my friends, and I'm running from God. I have such a good husband in Dan, and three children and a beautiful home—so much to be thankful for. But I'm so unhappy with myself!" And she obviously hated herself for being so out of control of her emotions.

"Ruth, I want to help you. And for heaven's sake, don't feel embarrassed about crying."

Ruth and Dan were newcomers to the church. She had always been friendly to me and was an enjoyable person to be around. I remembered the lovely lunch she had had, the day I had gotten to know Lois. Ruth had been the perfect hostess, making us feel right at home, and her home was beautiful and decorated with taste. Like Lois, Ruth was a teacher and did substitute work at the same school. She had been concerned about the project Lois had taken on at school and how involved it had become. I remember having the distinct feeling that Ruth really cared about Lois and me. I had never dreamed she was so unhappy inside.

But thinking about Lois reminded me of the good results she had had with a daily schedule. Maybe. . . .

"Ruth, ah, have you ever tried to specifically plan your days hour by hour?" I asked sheepishly.

"You mean some sort of a daily schedule?"

I was surprised she even had any idea what I was talking about. "Yes, that's exactly what I mean. If you planned your day with certain things at specific times, you might be less tempted to go back to bed." "Lois was telling me how much she had been helped by her new schedule," Ruth remarked. "And I can see a big change in her attitude and feelings about her house and family."

I couldn't help wondering, as Ruth talked, how a schedule would work out for her. She was not needy as far as her housework was concerned. She seemed to be able to keep a beautiful house and still have time for creativity—like flower arranging and needlepoint and things that added special touches to her home. But as she talked, her needs became more apparent. "I started making draperies and a bedspread for our bedroom two years ago, and they're not finished yet. And I have several other projects started, but not finished. I'd also like to get to know some women from church better, and I thought it would be fun to have a few small luncheons—I love to cook and entertain. But if I don't break this habit of running off to sleep every chance I get, none of those things can get done." She seemed to relax as we talked. Her eyes were puffy, red, and swollen from crying, but she was also at ease.

We just sat and talked for quite a while about a lot of different things. I found out that her husband was an engineer for the telephone company, and that they had been involved in a Methodist church before coming to Parkminster. Ruth started coming to the Wednesday morning Bible study with a neighbor, and loved it. Then she brought Dan a few times to hear guest speakers—and gradually she found herself spending more time at Parkminster than at her own church. Soon the whole family had joined in. By the time she got up to leave, I felt a real closeness to her— the very thing she had said she would not allow people to feel. It wasn't planned; it just happened. The sharing had broken down a self-constructed barrier. "I'm sure I look awful, but I feel better," she said, as she was getting ready to leave. "Thanks a lot—I'll need help to set up my schedule. Can we get together to work on it soon?" Schedule? I had already forgotten about working out her schedule. She went on, "Will it be all right if I call or stop in before the weekend? I want to start a new way of living Monday morning," she said with a big smile. "Sure, Ruth," I said, wondering when I was going to get the time on my own schedule to work on someone else's. I had Lois checking in with me, and now Ruth—who would be next?

I had mixed emotions when she drove out of the driveway. I knew it had been hard for her to come and share her need, and she was definitely being hurt by this bondage to sleep, but where would I find time? I decided I shouldn't get worried about it. God would have to stretch my days, that was all there was to it.

That night at supper Bill asked how my day had gone. I laughed and said, "Not on schedule, that's for sure." Then I told him about my morning visitors. "Sounds to me like God is answering our prayers about whether there should be a diet, discipline and discipleship group here," he laughed, "He sure seems to be making it obvious." "Well, let's quickly tell the Lord I'm willing, before I have ten more women coming one by one, asking to be put on schedules."

That very night I called Lois, Ruth, and Norma and shared the 3D idea with them. They thought it sounded tremendous and could think of several other women who would be interested in a group like this. So we set up a meeting time—the next Tuesday night at eight o'clock in the church lounge.

Tuesday night arrived—and so did ten women! Lois was the most enthusiastic of them all, with Ruth second. It was a funny group of people, some of us having never been together before.

I had invited Dee to come. She was a very heavy woman, a Catholic, who had called me on the phone one afternoon in reference to something I had written in my column in the local paper. I had talked with her several times since then and knew her weight problem was a big one. She needed help and was delighted that I had asked her to our meeting, even though she didn't know anyone there but me.

Then Lois had asked Margaret, who was in choir with her, and Mary Jane if they'd be interested. They were; both weighed over 200 pounds. Mary Jane had lost a lot of weight a few years back, but then gained it back again during a pregnancy.

The heavier women were obviously wondering why in the world Jo and Beverly were in the room. Neither of them weighed more than 120 pounds. I had asked them to come, not because they needed a diet group, but because I felt they could help us get some direction. They were both very active in Christian groups in the community with their husbands and seemed to lead very disciplined lives.

Then there was Norma, looking great from her dieting.

Helen came too. She had been in the Weight Watchers' group Dorcas and I had been part of; and like us, she had dropped out. We invited her to try 3D with some other "flunkies." And Dorcas reluctantly agreed to come too.

There was an uncomfortable silence in the room. Lois was busily introducing people to each other and still carrying the only real enthusiasm in the group. Dee seemed to be happy to meet these Protestant women. I knew I had to get the meeting started, even though I didn't have the slightest idea what we were going to do. The atmosphere was tense; the minute the talking stopped, I was scared. "I guess I should start off." I shared my ups and downs and ins and outs with this whole 3D idea, wanting it very desperately because of my own weight problem, and yet not willing to step out on faith to begin. "I'm ready now, with God's help, to see just what He has for us. Certainly, if the secular world can offer so much help to the over-indulger, God's got to have an even better answer. More and more I am seeing, and I think others are too, that our lives are totally undisciplined."

At this point, Lois jumped in. "This summer Carol helped me get myself on a daily schedule, with specific times to clean each room in my house, do my laundry and even play the piano and hike with the kids. We took a totally disorganized life, rearranged things with God's help, and it has literally changed my life in less than two months." She was radiant, sharing the blessings of the summer with the group.

MaryJane talked about how defeated she was, having gained all her weight back during her pregnancy. "I need help," she said rather desperately. She was a very attractive gal in her late twenties, but her weight was an obvious burden to her.

Norma spoke of her frustration with not being able to talk about God in her lectures at the diet group.

Jo and Beverly, the two who I thought would be able to guide us, confessed a lack of self-discipline in many areas of their lives. "Just because I'm not heavy doesn't mean I'm a disciplined person," Jo said. "I need help in a lot of ways." Beverly wholeheartedly concurred, and Ruth openly shared her struggle with sleeping too much. "Well," I announced, "here we are: the fat, the sleepy, and the sloppy, without a choice between us!" And we all roared with laughter. The tension in the air had pretty well vanished. We all agreed that we needed God's help and each other's help, and so we decided to meet every Tuesday night at eight, and just see what would happen.

The talking stopped, and someone suggested we pray before we leave. Spontaneously we stood up and joined hands in a circle. A spirit of quietness came over the room. An hour or so before, we had hardly known one another, but now, through sharing, we were becoming closer, God had been in our midst, and we all knew it.

Two Hearts are Better than One

"Where in the world have you been?" asked Bill drowsily, squinting at the clock. "Is that twenty minutes of twelve?"

I wished I hadn't bothered to turn on the light to get ready for bed. "I've been at the 3D meeting over at church," I replied, on my way to the bathroom. "Four hours at a 3D meeting? That doesn't sound very much like discipline to me!"

Shutting the bathroom door a little more forcefully than I'd intended, I began to rationalize why our fourth meeting had gone so late. Down inside, I was more upset about it than he was. But instead of telling him about my frustrations and getting it off my chest, I gave in to hurt feelings again and defended myself when I returned to the bedroom. "It was a bad week for all of us in the group, and we talked quite a bit about the problems we were having."

Bill didn't answer; he must have fallen back asleep. I reached over to shut off the lamp, somewhat relieved that he was sleeping, but also somewhat angry. After all, hadn't I often waited up for him when he came home late from church meetings? But the one night *I'm* late and really need to talk to him, he's asleep and only wakes up long enough to tell me I was wrong to be late! I punched my pillow, then scolded myself for being childish, but, as usual when I was in one of those moods, I ignored my own better judgment. Just then, almost as if he had heard my thoughts, Bill rolled over and grumbled, "Ten women should not be alone in the church so late at night, especially when they still have to drive home." And he rolled back over. "I never thought of that," I replied in a small voice, but there was no answer. Something else I never thought of was that the reasons I waited up for Bill were pretty selfish— usually I wanted to talk to him—and it didn't have a lot to do with my caring about him.

At that point I should have given the whole thing over to the Lord to resolve when and how He saw fit, and gone to sleep. Instead, I tossed and turned, thinking and churning it all around.

The group had been pretty good the first two weeks, even though we didn't seem to have much overall direction. The trouble was, we didn't know how to help each other, and we stopped short of saying what really needed to be said. For instance, I had felt that I should say something to Dee tonight about her three-pound gain, but how could I? I knew she was lonely and down because Sam, her husband, was out of town all week again, and besides, I had gained a pound and a half myself. I was also troubled to hear that Ruth had slept two or three afternoons, and I sensed that several of the others were troubled by that too. But all we did was say that it was sure better than sleeping five after-noons, like she used to. Jo hadn't been able to come at all because of another commitment, and I felt she was losing interest when I talked to her on the phone. And Helen was late. . . .

Oh, I wish I could forget the whole thing and go to sleep! But, of course, I couldn't. Like a gerbil on its exercise wheel, I started around again. Maybe this whole idea wasn't meant for us here in Rochester. Maybe. . . .

Only the face of the clock could be seen in our darkened bedroom. I tried to keep my eyes from it, hoping I'd fall asleep, but periodically I'd peek at it and almost watch the night and my precious sleep time, ticking away.

I started thinking again. It was bad enough that I myself had gained weight, but knowing four others had too really bothered me. It was easier in Weight Watchers, when I hadn't known the women personally. I paid no attention to their weight gains. What did they matter to me? But tonight was different. It really bothered me that Mary Jane and Helen had both recorded gains. And Lois certainly did not seem as positive and vibrant as she had at the beginning. And then I began to wonder what *they* were thinking about *me* tonight, their minister's wife not able to diet.

Around and around the exercise wheel went. I was sorry that I had ever heard those three words linked together—diet, discipline and discipleship. I'd much rather fight this diet thing alone than fail in front of nine other women. I looked at the clock; it was after three.

The next thing I knew, the alarm was ringing. It couldn't be 6:30; I didn't feel like I had slept at all! And in truth, I had been dreaming about 3D. The exercise wheel had gone right on turning in my sleep; no wonder I felt so exhausted. I managed to get out of bed and wander downstairs to start breakfast and make school lunches. Bill came down thirty minutes later. "Well, late one?" he said. "I'll bet you're good and tired this morning." And he went to the door, to get the morning paper. He was smiling, but it made me angry all over again, and I bit my lip to keep from replying the way I wanted to. Instead, I admitted that I had been awake half the night—disturbed about the 3D meeting, trying to solve all the problems of the group by myself.

Bill let me wind down, and then said simply, "Sounds to me like you need some leadership in that group, if for no other reason than to end it after an hour or so." He sat down and turned to the sports page. "You can't just wander around in each other's problems for four hours and then go home and expect to get a good night's sleep," he remarked from behind the paper.

Ouch! He had hit right on target and in five seconds come up with what had eluded me half the night. But I could already sense what was coming next, and I wanted no part of it! "If you're suggesting that I lead that group, the answer is no. I need help in discipline desperately—and in diet! Besides, I've led enough things in that church! It's someone else's turn!" I got up quickly and started clearing the table. He hadn't said one word about my leading the group, but I knew what he was thinking. I yanked the dishwasher door open and jerked the top rack out.

"I wonder if the reason the Cape Cod group went so well," Bill asked gently, "was because of the leadership Jane and Lenny brought to it?" "I'm sure it did. They certainly knew something about what they were doing," I retorted. "And you know the disciplined lives they lead at the Community. That would make a great deal of difference in leading a group. "Pray about it, Carol," Bill said simply. "Jane and Lenny would be the first to tell you that *God* made the group work at that Cape Cod church, not their nutrition or diet expertise.

You know, it could be God's will, and you need to stay open to that possibility." He turned to the editorial page. I said nothing. But I was so mad that it was a miracle I didn't break a plate, putting it in the dishwasher. And what made me even madder was that I sensed he was right—again.

We didn't talk any more about 3D after that morning session, and I did my best to forget the whole discussion in the days that followed. There was never a lack of things to do at home or at church, so I just wrapped myself up in the various needs around me. The week slipped by, and soon it was Tuesday again. Just the thought that we might end up talking until midnight made me want to skip the 3D meeting entirely. But I knew I had no choice.

It was a beautiful clear October evening, with a nip in the air foretelling the onset of winter. In the yard the trees were an array of color—copper and gold and deep red. The children had raced outside, as soon as dinner was over, to get a little more playtime in before bedtime. Peter had his yellow Tonka trucks moving the earth around; Betsy had an old pink blanket spread out with dolls and stuffed animals all over it, having a family picnic. Tim was riding his bike around the house.

Just as I was ready to walk across the yard to church, my dad and my brother Brian drove in. I was delighted. What a perfect excuse not to go to the 3D meeting! My father had retired the previous year and moved to Rochester to live close to us. Brian, thirteen, was my "little" brother. He often seemed more like a son to us, and an older brother to the children. Unfortunately, my mother's premature death and my Dad's job transfer made it necessary for Brian to live with us until Dad could take an early retirement. As soon as Dad moved to Rochester and found a little apartment with Brian, just a mile and a half down the road, they became part of our family and dropped in all the time. "Hi, Sis!" Brian yelled out the open window, "Where are you going?" "Oh, I was just going to some meeting at church, but I'd love to visit with you and Dad instead," I said, turning and starting to walk towards their car. "We're not coming to visit," Brian replied quickly. "We just wanted to know if the kids wanted to go for a swim before bed."

We had a family swim membership over at the Sheraton Motel, and the children were able to swim there twelve months a year in the enclosed pool. "Oh, please, Mom, *please,* can we go?" Betsy pleaded, jumping up and down with excitement, totally forgetting about her doll's family picnic on the blanket. "Me, too! I want to go swim with Brian," Peter yelled and ran over to the car, grabbing Brian's outstretched arm.

Dad didn't even bother to shut the engine off. We chatted while the kids raced in to get towels and swimsuits. In no time, they were out again, piling into the back seat, and off they went, waving. And with them went my excuse for skipping 3D.

I was late. Hurrying across the yard, I slipped into the church and up the stairs to the little chapel. We had decided the week before to move into the chapel, where we could have some privacy. Situated in the middle of the church, the library tended to be a high traffic zone. People who wanted to go into the church office had to go through the library; people who were counseling with Bill usually waited in the library; and anyone heading towards the choir loft or the sanctuary had to pass through there too.

I opened the chapel door, and found I was the last one to arrive. "Oh," Ruth remarked, "I thought you

might be at the preschool meeting downstairs tonight."
"Preschool meeting? Oh my goodness, I forgot!" I said, clapping my hand over my mouth. I had just finished my term as chairman of the committee, and I was easing my way out, but I was expected to be there tonight. Preschool—there was the perfect excuse for not staying at 3D tonight. But now that I was here, I knew I couldn't run out on them. "I'll go down in a little while after we share," I said. "The preschool meetings are always late in finishing anyway." "Speaking of finishing late," Mary Jane remarked, "my John thinks *these* meetings go much too late. He finally drove the babysitter home at 11:15 last week and had to leave the children unattended. That didn't make him very happy, and he said he hoped that didn't happen again tonight!"

So Bill wasn't the only one. Helen and Ruth, too, were concerned about the same thing. And then Margaret spoke up. "You know, we might as well face it: What we really need for the group is a leader." "I agree," Dee chimed in. "And the other problem we have," Ruth stated, "is that no one wants to really speak up. I didn't get the help I needed last week, and I didn't help anyone else, I'm afraid. And what good is a group like that?" she asked bluntly.

Most of the others in the group were nodding and murmuring their assent. "Someone to lead would be a big help," Helen agreed. I glanced over at Dorcas, but she wasn't saying a word; in her own way, she was as resistant as I was. For she, too, could read the handwriting on the wall. A long, very uncomfortable silence fell over the group.

Norma broke it, as several eyes fell on her. "I wish I could lead this group," she said apologetically, "but there's no way I can. I signed an agreement with my other diet group, that I would not lead any other group for at least six months after I finished with them."

I had hoped Norma was the answer for us, but now that was out. "How about you, Dorcas?" I asked. "You're a teacher and a good one; you could do a great job." "You've got to be kidding! Me, the big flunky from every weight-watching group in town, leading a diet group? It will be a major accomplishment for me just to stay in this group until the end of the program." She laughed. And then everyone else laughed with her, and that broke the tension. Someone suggested we pray about who should lead. A great idea, I thought; why hadn't it occurred to me?

But, before we could pray, Lois said, "Carol, as the senior minister's wife, aren't you the most likely one to lead the group?" "Lois," I replied, so vehemently that I startled myself, as well as the others, "I'm *tired* of leading groups! Let someone else lead for a change."

The tenseness returned to the room, and I knew it was my fault. My attitude was lousy. Feeling a little sheepish about it, I said, "I guess we'd better ask God to help us to know His will about this."

All of us knew, of course, that God had to make the difference in this group. If He didn't, we might as well join all the other diet and self-help groups in the community. I felt chagrined that we had not gone to Him first.

There was quite a bit of silent prayer, then a few audible prayers. I'm not sure how long this prayer time went on, but something was happening to me during it. I was softening. I knew I had to give up my resistance and be willing to lead this group. Someone else prayed, "God, show us Your will, and then help us to do it."

After that prayer time, the way seemed very clear. The group asked me to lead, and I was pleased to say yes. And Dorcas said she was also willing to lead, if needed, which meant her heart had been changed too. We decided to try to lead the group as a team of two. This way, there would be an added check and balance, as two hearts were often better at hearing the Holy Spirit than one. Dual leadership was also being tried around us, both in public school education and in Sunday school. That sounded super to me. So, in spite of our discouragement and resistance as a group, God moved us on. The leaders were ready, the group was enthusiastic, and we were all aware of God's presence and direction in a new way.

We decided that our meetings should last only one hour. We would all weigh in before meeting time and start right at eight We also agreed to pray for each member of the group every day. Mary Jane volunteered to type up a prayer list for us with names and telephone numbers.

Just about then, I happened to notice the chapel doorknob turn slowly, and the door open just a crack. Looking carefully, I thought I could see Bill, glancing in. "Come on in," I said, motioning with my hand. "We've had a great time tonight." "Are you almost ready to go home?" he said with a big smile. "Or are you going to stay on until midnight again?" "We are getting so organized, you won't believe us," Dorcas answered. "You're right, I won't believe you," he laughed heartily.

He wasn't at all surprised to learn that Dorcas and I were "elected" to be group leaders. "I sort of felt that that was the direction you should take," he admitted. That breakfast-table scene last week flashed through my mind at that moment. Bill winked at me.

He shared with the group his enthusiasm for their undertaking and felt it was an area of great need in the church. "There's a verse that says that discipline is painful for the moment but that later it will produce the fruit of righteousness." He looked up at our blank faces. "It's in Hebrews," he said, picking up the Bible on the altar. "Here, Hebrews 12:11."

I had read the book of Hebrews several times, but somehow I felt as though I was hearing that verse for the first time. And judging from the reactions of the others, they felt the same way.

Beverly made a suggestion: "Why don't we memorize a verse of Scripture every week?"

I swallowed hard. I had not been able to memorize Scripture since I was a young girl in Sunday school. And a quick glance around the room indicated I wasn't alone.

She suggested we start with the verse Bill had just quoted.

"It will be a big help to us, as we try to be more disciplined as a group."

Bill agreed wholeheartedly. "There are many things all through the Bible that talk about our need for leading disciplined lives, that God might be glorified in our bodies." He flipped through the pages, stopping here and there and reading a few verses. "Would you be willing," I asked him, "to come in every week just for a few minutes, to share things like that with us?" "Sure."

The end of a perfect evening. We felt like a real group now, adventuring together on a new path. And having Bill come in made us feel a part of the church instead of just a bunch of women meeting at church. God was having His way after all.

SEVEN

TRUSTING

I felt excited and happy now as Tuesday evenings approached. I even looked forward to leading the group, and I sensed that much of the change in my attitude was directly attributable to the daily prayer—both mine for all the others in the group, and theirs for me. Our mutual commitment had turned out to be a lot harder than any of us expected; it was also producing unexpected results. None of us had had very much practice in laying aside our own cares and concerns in order to fully concentrate on the needs of others, even for only a few minutes a day. But we were beginning to get the hang of it.

At first, I had resented the prospect of coming to know the other women's failures. I felt my own were enough for me to cope with; I did not want the responsibility of having to care about others, too. But I soon became deeply convicted of what an ugly attitude this was—about as far from Christ's as it was possible to get. And never mind spiritualizing it; I knew plenty of non-Christians who cared more about other people than I did.

I was sorry. I determined to care enough to take their needs to God, which was the very best care I could give.

God did not expect me to heal their weaknesses or carry their burdens. But He did expect me to take their needs to Him. And what's more, they were doing the same thing with my needs. We were all part of a team, working together, to get our lives more under the control of God. It was not a chore but a privilege.

We were learning a great deal in a hurry—not points of doctrine, but practical ways to put our faith in God to work in the most mundane things of daily life. It became more and more apparent to me that my Christianity still revolved almost entirely around me, rather than around Christ. Oh, of course, I brought the big things of my life to Him. But the little things—the shopping list, the order of the day's priorities—were still my domain. I did things my way and in my time, and God had very little to do with them. What did things like the way I made the beds each day, or cooked the meals, or sewed on buttons, have to do with God? He certainly had much bigger things in the world to be concerned about.

And yet I knew from the Bible that every hair on my head was numbered, and that not a sparrow fell to the ground without the Father in heaven being aware of it. I had always accepted those facts in my head, but I had no idea how to translate them into my life.

Now I was beginning to see that if He cared about the sparrow's fall, He would be interested in my shopping list. The small, personal concerns of my life and the greatness of God's love were finally coming together. The smallest, most insignificant details of my daily life were opportunities to glorify Him. Imagine eating, sewing, cooking, and cleaning house to the glory of God!

Along with this new awareness, I was now becoming convicted of my disobedience in little things. The still, small voice that I had successfully ignored so many times by telling myself that God couldn't possibly care about such small details, was becoming louder and dearer all the time. He *did* care—I was the one who didn't.

As I listened more closely now, I began to see how my family meals were cooked and planned according to how I happened to feel at the moment, instead of according to what He might want, or to His glory. For instance, if I happened to feel super, I would bake some pumpkin pie or chocolate chip cookies, or broil some steaks or make some homemade French fries. But if I didn't feel like bothering, then tuna casserole or Sloppy Joes would do just fine. God was showing me how unloving this was and how it not only gypped my family but also failed to glorify Him. I had to stop doing things so uncaringly and selfishly and start doing things to please God.

As this whole idea of doing even the littlest things to the glory of God—that is, *living* for Him—became clearer in my mind, I began to see why I had been so uncomfortable in my previous diet group. The emphasis of that group had been to help me become a better *me!* I dieted so I could wear nicer clothes, get more attention from my husband and family, and have a good self-image. It was me at the center, but the center of my life was supposed to be God.

The old way had worked. I felt a hundred percent better, I bought new clothes, my husband loved the new me, and people at church and everywhere else raved about how wonderful I looked. But where did God fit into all of this? He didn't! It was an ego trip—a self-glorifying experience that, if I was interested in drawing closer to God, was exactly what I did not need.

The main problem, of course, was not with the weight-watching program; it was with me. I had always thrived on the attention of others. In fact, I felt, deep down, that I couldn't live without it. In high school I was a drum majorette, now I was a minister's wife. All kinds of ups and downs in my life could be explained by the amount of attention and acceptance I was enjoying. But it was a trap.

I was finally beginning to understand that my acceptance had to be found in God—not in how I looked or what I weighed. And if I was convicted that my willful self-indulgence in the food department and my refusal to say no to self were not pleasing to God, then I should change for that reason, not for vanity's sake or the sake of a better self-image.

But the fact that the picture was clearer to me now didn't make it any easier. It was still just as hard to resist a piece of banana cream pie. And it still wasn't easy to discipline myself to pray every day for the group members. It would generally take only ten minutes or so to go down the prayer list, but I was finding that I couldn't stay with God for even that long, to intercede for the needs of others. Like a willful little child, my mind would persist in wandering off to what I had to do that day. God had obviously brought 3D into my life for more reasons than dieting.

How thankful I was for that time, a year before, when Cay and Judy had suggested that I consider assuming a three-month discipline of not criticizing Bill. That was what it had taken to break my obnoxious and ultimately destructive habit of pick, pick, pick, that was pervading our marriage and home. For me, that had been the forerunner of the whole 3D concept. I reminded myself that three months had been a very small price to pay for what had happened. So when it was tough to stick to these new disciplines, I would remind myself of how free I now felt because of the disciplines the previous May. And I'd go on— expecting the same sort of change to take place in me.

Others in the group were also struggling, but as we shared together on Tuesday nights, I found that they, too, were learning about the blessings of being disciplined. And, not only were we learning together, we were enjoying just being together. Our hour together on Tuesday nights didn't seem nearly long enough any more. On Sunday mornings after the church service, we would gather around in the narthex and catch up on each other's diets or sewing or house projects. Nor was it unusual to answer the phone and hear, "Hi, this is Helen. I couldn't wait until Tuesday to tell you what happened to me today!" In these few months together, a bond of love in Christ was being established among us. It was easy now to call and ask one of the others for special prayer; we were not ashamed to be needy and share our most seemingly foolish problems. For example, whom else could one call to ask for prayer that one not eat the Swiss chocolate almond ice cream in the freezer while everyone was out of the house?

There had been very few people in our church with whom I had ever shared much of myself. I had an image of what a good minister's wife should be, and a part of that image was to be able to handle small problems myself—like dieting and cleaning house. I was sure they would not be interested in all my petty grievances or even understand that those things would bother me. But I was wrong. Just the opposite was true. As I shared my personal needs, the women felt much closer to me.

One of them confessed one night in the group that she had been scared to death of sharing her small needs in front of "the minister's wife" for fear she would be rejected. But she lost her fear when she heard I had some of the same feelings. We laughed together and saw how silly all of this was, and what ridiculous images we had of one another. After that, I wondered if it wasn't indeed one of the Devil's ways of keeping Christians from getting too close to one another, to let them believe they would be unacceptable to one another if the truth about themselves were known.

New relationships were springing up within our group every week. Mary Jane told one night of how she had judged me two years before, because of an episode with the Christian education committee. They had asked me to teach the senior high Sunday school class and had assigned me a topic, giving me specific materials to use. I had not been comfortable with the materials and had requested permission to use something else. "I was furious that you would dare question the material we had picked out," Mary Jane recalled. "After all, I was a school teacher, and you weren't. What right did you have to override our decision?" She paused, and shook her head at the memory. "From that night on, I decided I really didn't like you, even if you were the new minister's wife." "Wow," I said, awed by this confession, "and I never even realized anything was wrong. You've always been pleasant to me." "Oh, yes, pleasant, but not really friendly," she said, laughing. "But now, since I've been in this group with you and praying for you every day, I feel totally different. Please forgive me for holding such a silly grudge against you all this time."

I went over and threw my arms around her and gave her a big hug. She threw her arms around me, and there we stood, both of us laughing and wiping tears from our eyes at the same time.

After that we were more open and honest than ever. We talked about our buried grudges and resentments. Many of us had kidded ourselves that they didn't matter anyway, but deep down we knew that these things did seriously affect our relationships with others. So, by the gentle leading of the Holy Spirit, we were finding healing and renewal.

Dee deeply resented Sam's job, which required him to be out of town so much. And there seemed to be a clear connection between that anger and the hard time she had with her weight. "When I'm lonely, I eat—and especially at night after the children go to bed." she admitted. And several of the women in the group encouraged her to call them when she felt like that— before she ate the chocolate cake or dish of ice cream. And each of us could pray a lot more specifically for Dee after that.

Beverly, who tended to be very quiet and rather standoffish, told about how hurt she had been as a young girl when her mother died. "I guess, way back there, I decided that I'd better just pull back from people and make it on my own and not get too close to anyone again!" she said.

Just that little bit of sharing from Bev made us all feel closer to her. We were all beginning to see that these small, seemingly insignificant things were prevalent in all of us and did indeed affect our relationships with one another. It was as though we were all imprisoned in invisible, solitary confinement cells, afraid to reveal ourselves beyond the most superficial level. And yet, when we did, the love of God and the caring that poured out among us were incredible!

The 3D meetings got better every week Now everyone was being open, and the flow of the Spirit in the group seemed really good. And then, one night in early

December, Bill dropped what, to me, felt like a one-ton bomb. He asked us if we thought we were reaching out enough to others. "Yes, like never before!" one of the group exclaimed, and several others quickly agreed. Bill listened, as we then took turns expounding on the ways we had reached out to one another.

Suddenly he cut across the testimony. "I'm delighted with what's happening in the group, but what about outside of the group?"

Gulp. I wasn't thinking about beyond the group. I was just so glad to see what was happening in the group. For crying out loud! What does he expect in just three months? "Have you invited other women in the church who have some of the same problems you do, to join your group?" he asked pointedly.

That made me mad! But I bit my lip, and decided to wait until I got home to let him know how I felt. I wasn't about to expose my anger in front of the group—I couldn't be *that* honest!

There was an uncomfortable silence for several moments. Then Helen quietly spoke up, a sense of conviction in her voice: "I'm sure you are picking up something that we need to face up to." She took a deep breath and went on. "I can see that it would be very easy to get comfortable in this group and even become a clique—but we can't afford to. We are only a very small part of Parkminster's women, and there are lots more than ourselves we need to be concerned about."

Dee spoke next. "I've often felt funny about being a part of this group, when I don't even belong to your church. And I've had the thought that there might be women in this church who deserved to be a part of this group, instead of me." "Don't feel that way, Dee!" I blurted out. "We're glad to have you as a part of this group, and it doesn't matter a bit that you go to another church." Brother, was I going to say a few things to Bill when I got home!

But for some reason the rest of the group didn't seem nearly as upset as I was; in fact, I was shocked at their positive response to what he was saying. "As much as I hate the thought of having the group change or enlarge," Lois said, "I think we really do have to think about others in the church who might want to be a part of this group. And without thinking very hard, I can come up with three or four friends who I know would join tomorrow if they could."

"Scares me, too," Ruth confessed, "and I'm afraid we might lose the closeness and trust we've found over these months. But I guess we'll have to trust God again, won't we?"

Bill nodded approvingly. "I understand your apprehension, but I believe it is time to invite others. God has been changing your lives—more than you ever expected, and in a remarkably short time, when you stop to think about it. And it happened because you've trusted Him and have been obedient to what He's required of you. But now you need to share that. He won't stop working just because the group gets bigger. Remember, He is a very big God!"

The others laughed at that, but I was still smoldering inside at the mere thought of a change in the group. And Dorcas, I noticed, was conspicuously silent also; I was sure she felt as I did.

Finally I had to speak. "Well, you've certainly given us something to think about, and we will. But with the holidays practically on top of us, we probably won't have time to really consider it until after the New Year."

But Bill would not be put off. "I think after the New Year is when you should begin with new members, not just consider it."

At this point I gladly could have shouted at him, yet somehow I kept silent and even kept smiling. But just wait till we got home. . . .

Dorcas broke the tense silence. "Well, speaking for myself, it seems to me that we have considered it tonight, and, frankly, I feel that we are supposed to do something about it—now. I know I've been convicted by what Bill has said to us."

Dorcas! I looked at her, feeling almost betrayed. But with my own emotions so obviously distraught, I decided I'd better leave the rest of the plans and discussion to the others. I sat through it all, but was withdrawn, trying to figure out why I was reacting so to this suggestion. I had begun to calm down inside, and now I was shocked at the violence of my initial reaction.

I was relieved when the meeting broke up; I needed to get in touch with what was happening deep within me, and I sensed it was something I wasn't to bring up in the whole group. So instead of going home, I decided to wait in the church library to see if I might see Bill between his counseling appointments. I needed some counseling pretty badly myself.

Confused, I began to seek the Lord's help. And for no apparent reason, all of a sudden I found myself thinking about our former church in Bridgeport. And then a specific scene came to mind: it was our last morning in Bridgeport. Our furniture had already left for Rochester, and we were spending the night at a parishioner's home. I woke up almost before it was dawn outside and was suddenly overcome with inexplicable grieving. It made no sense at all. I knew we were in God's will to move; we'd said our goodbyes and were looking forward to our new church. But suddenly I was so overcome with the thought of leaving, that I just sat on my side of the bed and sobbed. I had my hand over my mouth, but I woke Bill anyway. "What's the matter, hon, can't you sleep anymore?" "Sleep? Who can sleep when we are about to leave the people we love so much!" I cried. "And it doesn't seem to bother you at all—don't you have any feelings?"

Apparently sensing that nothing he could say would help, he came over and sat next to me, put his arm around me and let me cry it out on his shoulder.

What a curious thing to think of, after all these years! And then I saw the connection: I was having the same kinds of feelings tonight, just thinking about changing the makeup of our 3D group. In an instant, I saw how much I put my security in relationships—first at Bridgeport and now in the 3D group—and how comparatively little in Christ. Tied in with my fear of rejection, this situation felt explosive to me. Acceptance meant everything to me, and now here was a group that accepted me—overweight and undisciplined—a group that I could really be *me* in, and now it was being taken from me.

It wasn't all clear to me, and I was anxious for Bill's help in putting the pieces in place, but as I waited for his door to open I became aware of another grief— only this one was not my own. For the first time in my life, I thought of how Jesus must feel, and must have felt all these years, as I consistently turned to others for my security instead of to Him. Now I *really* had something to feel sorry about!

By the time Bill finished his appointment, my anger had dissipated, and I was a little sheepish at what had happened earlier. When I shared it all with Bill, he was surprised at first to hear that the whole Bridgeport thing had surfaced again but quickly saw the same connection. "God has been trying for a long time to get you to put your trust in Him. But He's also been patiently waiting for you to reach a place where you would be ready. You're ready now."

EIGHT

A New Beginning

Christmas season 1973 came on us quickly, and the activities were in full swing both around the house and the church. All of our holiday schedules were such that we had decided not to meet for 3D again until the first Tuesday of the new year. As much as I missed the fellowship of the group, I was grateful to have one less meeting to go to. There was so much to do: In addition to our family's preparation, there were the church's needs—decorating, planning carol sings, baking cookies and breads, making food baskets for shut-ins, and producing special pageants by the various youth groups. And then no sooner would Christmas be over, than plans and preparations would begin for the big New Year's Eve dinner and service at church.

In our household the traditional sign that the season was upon us was when Bill and the children went on their annual Christmas tree expedition. And back they would come, with the biggest and fullest tree they could find tied to the top of our station wagon. This year, as usual, Bill had been too extravagant, and at least a foot would have to be chopped off the top; in fact, the branches had to be trimmed before it would fit through the front door! But I had to admit that I, too, loved a full Christmas tree, and so I put out of mind the thought of all those pine needles in the living room carpet for months after Christmas, and joined in.

While Bill and the children lugged the big boxes of decorations down from the attic, I began selecting the Christmas Hummels from the bookcase shelves— shelves high up, out of the reach of little hands, for these delicate figures had become very special to me over the years. The soft, hand-painted features made them just perfect for Christmas scenes. I loved especially the figures of Mary and the Baby Jesus. She was kneeling with her arms spread, as if to say, "See, my Son, the Holy One of God," and her eyes were closed in thanks to her heavenly Father. The Baby Jesus lay on the hay with a white cloth under him; his eyes were open and bright, his hands responding to his mother's presence. Beside his bed, I placed the little figure of a sheep, which watched Him intently, its eyes fixed on the bed and its ears sticking out, listening. In my collection I had only two kings, and these I placed just off to one side at a respectful distance. One, a black man with a turban and footwear that laced halfway up his legs, stood with one hand on his sword, and the other holding out a gift of frankincense. The second king was an older man, with a beard and a crown-shaped hat. He was kneeling, offering a little chest of gold to the mother and child. Surrounding the manger scene, I put little angels playing musical instruments. And once the last angel was in place, I straightened up and surveyed the scene. Now let the celebration begin!

To a weak-willed glutton, Christmas is an endless procession of goodies—fancy cookies, spiced punch bowls, rich creamy eggnog, and cranberry breads! It was customarily impossible for me to diet over the holidays; gaining weight seemed as much a part of the holiday season as getting a Christmas tree. But somehow I had the feeling of its being different this year; the battle seemed easier. And I knew that the extra will power I now seemed to have was coming out of the group; for even though we were not meeting together, there were still nine friends praying for me every day.

In fact, everything was going beautifully over the holidays—until the Sunday after Christmas. I was sitting in church, waiting for the service to begin and looking over the bulletin, when one announcement jumped out at me.

> Any women who might be interested in joining the group that has been dealing with problems of diet, discipline and discipleship should meet in the chapel on Tuesday, January 7, at 8 pm.

With a jolt I realized that I had completely put out of mind the reality that our group was going to be enlarged the next time we met. Never again would it just be the ten of us. And sure enough, just thinking about it brought up again those same feelings of fear and betrayal and—but the difference was that now I recognized them and could turn them right over to the Lord before I went down under them. So I prayed, "Jesus, help me now," and set my will to trust Him, and to be obedient to His leading. Once I had done that, I felt peace return, and it remained through the rest of the service.

✍

January 7th, 7:45 PM: A dozen chairs in the little chapel had been removed from the neat rows facing the altar and arranged into a small circle. The old "3Ders" had arrived early for a quick weight check-in.

The news was bad but not awful for most of us—two or three pounds up—and not nearly as bad as it had been in previous years, for which we were all rejoicing. There was a warm feeling amongst us. "Looks like three weeks off is just a little more than most of us disciplined dieters can handle," Dee called toward the scale that was located in the east hall. "That's for sure," I called back, marking my two-pound gain on the old chart. "Boy, have I missed the group," Helen said, "and more than just to check my weight!" "Me, too," remarked Dee. "And I didn't see any of you during the holidays." She had worked hard at St. Helen's Catholic Church over the holidays.

As we waited for the newcomers, we took turns telling what had been happening without diets and disciplines since last we met. Though most of us had seen each other fairly frequently at the holiday events, it never seemed appropriate to bring up 3D. Yet now we laughed and talked together as if we had never been apart. We had left the chapel door ajar, half watching for newcomers, but having really forgotten that they were coming. All of a sudden the door opened, and a voice interrupted us. "Is this where the diet and discipline group is meeting?"

I looked towards the door. It was Judith! What in the world was she doing here? She was stunning—tall, slender and stylish. "Yes, Judith," I managed, "come on in," and I tried to smile encouragingly to conceal my dismay.

Three more women followed closely behind. All four of them looked as though they could have stepped out of fashion magazines. The warmth that had been flowing through the chapel moments before was gone, and in its place, a chill of lack of trust settled over the room.

Mary Jane offered to get more chairs to enlarge the circle, and as more newcomers arrived, we needed five, then ten, and then twenty. Women were filing in at an unbelievable pace, one right after another, and before long the circle was touching the altar rail at one end of the room and the folding doors at the other. When some really fat women finally joined the circle, I felt a little guilty to be so delighted to see them. But for a few minutes there, it had looked as if the thin ones were going to take over 3D.

I was astounded at the turnout; by eight o'clock there were thirty-nine women in the room! We squeezed together closely, many keeping their winter coats on and pocket books in their laps, making the circle seem even tighter. There was a strained, uncomfortable atmosphere in the room; I could sense the feelings that were floating around—fear, anxiety, jealousy, and more than a little judgment.

A hush fell over the group a few minutes after eight, and all eyes turned towards me. I was speechless, even prayerless, but I finally managed a "Jesus, help me!" under my breath. Then I had no choice but to trust Him and begin to talk.

First. I shared about my experience in the nationally known diet group. That seemed to crack the ice a little, and looking around I recognized several women whom I had seen attending those meetings. But there was still a strong "Okay, show me" attitude in the room. My hands were clasped in my lap, and I was twisting my engagement ring around and around on my finger. My hand was stone cold, so my ring moved freely and probably could have fallen off without too much effort. "Unfortunately," I went on, "soon after I had reached my weight goal and graduated, the pounds slowly began to creep back on. Nor was this the first time—in fact, it was a depressing pattern of mine—that long months of painful dieting were wiped away in just a few weeks. And as before, I had promised myself that this time it would be different. After all, I had become quite learned about calories and carbohydrates, and just which foods did what. But all the head knowledge I possessed was powerless when it came up against my strong determination to indulge myself." The group knew exactly what I was talking about, and several heads were nodding around the circle.

"Something was missing from my experience in the diet group. It had been a tremendous help to me—I did lose thirty-seven pounds! But, when I went back to rejoin last May, something inside of me balked. I just couldn't do it." I had the feeling that others in this group had experienced the same thing, and that perhaps that was why they were here tonight. "And then God spoke to me through a red smile-face painted on a Sunday school partition. The words under the face said, 'Smile, God has the answer.' And He did, though it was nearly a year before He showed it to me."

I went on briefly to tell about the start of 3D and also about the positive impression I had of the disciplined life in the Community of Jesus. "I knew I was undisciplined and not just in the area of food. What I saw on Cape Cod seemed to me to somehow contain the answer."

Abruptly the words ran out. I stopped, not knowing what else to say. Dorcas smoothly picked up the discussion and went on. As she got into what she was saying, I was again aware of what a blessing it was to have two leaders instead of one. Way back when God had practically forced the two of us to become co-leaders, I had had no idea how it was going to turn out, but how many times I had been grateful since—like tonight. For one thing, no meeting depended all on one person. When the flow of words dried up for one of us, it seemed as if the other leader, was just ready to start. God had known what He was doing that night, and here I had thought it was only because we were both so resistant!

"I have joined and quit more diet groups and spent more money trying to lose weight in the past year than probably anyone else in this room!" Dorcas exclaimed, to a ripple of knowing laughter. Apparently she was not the only one in the join-quit category. "I kept thinking I could do it myself, once I had gotten a little start from a group, but it never worked for more than a few weeks. Yet, during these past ten or twelve weeks, something has been happening in me. I've begun to understand that it is part of God's plan that we help one another, instead of being so determined to do it ourselves. And that has put dieting in a whole new ballpark for me."

As the two of us continued, back and forth, illustrating from our own experiences, what tension remained in the room perceptibly relaxed. "I have come to admit and recognize that I am an undisciplined person," I concluded. "The 3D group has been a real help to my life in Christ. I am learning for the first time how to really *care* for someone else besides myself." There, I had said it! Openly and honestly. And it felt good.

We opened the meeting for a time of sharing then, and what a blessing that turned out to be! There was no pretense, no phoniness, just honesty. Ruth told of her unfinished draperies and bedspread, and lots of the women could identify with her. "They had been sitting around our bedroom for two years waiting to be finished, and during the weeks I was in 3D, I finished them! So you can imagine how delighted my husband was to see them on the windows and on the bed instead of in a corner of the bedroom. The prayers and support of the 3D group did it—I just know they did."

Mary Jane spoke next. "I haven't done that great in the weight department, but lots else has happened to me. I didn't know any of the women in this group very well, and those I did know, I didn't particularly like." Several laughed at her candor. "But when you pray for someone every day, your petty gripes disappear. Before I knew it, not only did I like them all, but God gave me a real love for them—His love." Tears filled her eyes, and her voice broke. "I just can't tell you how different I feel," she concluded, smiling.

I felt tears welling up in my own eyes and saw them in a number of others' eyes as well. Helen got up and went to get a box of Kleenex, leaving the chapel door open to relieve the stuffiness of the small room. That helped to relax the group even more, although almost all the tension had already lifted. She came back and handed the Kleenex box to Mary Jane, who passed it on.

Then Ann Marie spoke up. "When can I become a part of this group?" "Well—" I started, not knowing quite how to answer. "This is an answer to prayer to me," Ann Marie added. "I *need* a group like this."

I knew Ann Marie from working with her on the preschool committee. She took a very active role in the church, although her husband was not involved at all. "I'm ready to start in a group like this tomorrow," she said and sat down.

And indeed there was a definite feeling in the room of "Let's get on with it." Dorcas and I looked at one another, a little amazed. "How many of you feel, like Ann Marie, that a group like this is something you are really interested in?" I asked. Every single hand went up! "But you haven't even heard what we do in the group, or what disciplines are required." "Maybe after they hear the requirements, they won't be quite as interested!" Dorcas said with a smile. "First," I said, drawing myself up to my most imposing posture, "you have to be on time for every meeting. In fact, you have to come fifteen minutes before the scheduled time, in order to get weighed in. And everyone must weigh in, weight problem or not. Also, you must commit yourself to come every week, unless, of course, there is a genuine emergency for you." Still no resistance in the room.

Dorcas took it from there. "We have also made a commitment to one another to pray at a specific time each day without fail for everyone else in the group." With this, she held up a copy of our prayer list, so everyone could see it. "Praying for one another has changed every one of our attitudes as dramatically as Mary Jane's."

Marilyn, a petite woman weighing not more than a hundred pounds, brought up a concern. "I've come tonight because I need help in my spiritual life. But I'm sitting here wondering how I am ever going to find time to pray for thirty-nine women every day, when I can't find time to pray for my four children!"

I smiled, because that same thought had crossed my mind just a few moments before. "I don't really know, Marilyn. We never dreamed we'd have this many here tonight. God will have to show us how it is going to work."

I took a fresh look around the circle. There were Sue, a very attractive young mother and a newcomer to the church; Jan, a rather stocky, pretty woman who was a head nurse at Strong Memorial Hospital; Barbara, the new church secretary; and other familiar faces. I knew their names, but I felt as though I hardly knew them beyond that. Suddenly, I felt as if I was on the brink of knowing them better and letting them know me better, and that felt good to me.

But how was it all going to work? Bill and I talked about it after the meeting that night, and neither of us felt right about just having one, great big group. The openness and trust had just begun in the small group of ten, and it definitely seemed that this was what God wanted for us. We both agreed that it was indeed God's direction, and He had blessed it, so we'd better stay with it and have two or three small groups, instead of one big one. "But who is going to lead if we have three groups?" I asked. "Guess," Bill said with a half smile. "Oh. . . . How in the world will we ever find the time?" I groaned. "Well, remember, 3D is God's idea," he laughed, "so He'll just have to make more time for you and Dorcas."

NINE

"I Want to be Myself!"

From January 1974 until the end of March, there were three diet, discipline and discipleship groups meeting in the church every week. Beverly helped Dorcas and me with the leadership responsibilities, filling in and replacing either of us when necessary, which was often enough so that we really counted on her.

One of the first things we invested in was a big hospital-type scale for weighing in. Although the cost was well over a hundred dollars, there was no problem raising the money from the members of the groups. In fact, it was even suggested that we take a weekly offering to purchase the things we might need, though there was little that was necessary for a diet group beyond an accurate scale! Now there could be no more shaving a pound or two by shifting towards the right front or leaning towards the back left corner. Every quarter of a pound would register, no matter what you did! Naturally, everyone was excited at first with a new, highly accurate scale, but in the weeks to come there were more than a few of us who occasionally wished for our old bathroom standby back!

At one of the evening groups, I was busy marking the weight chart as everyone came in, when I noticed that Barbara had slipped in and not said a word about her weight.

"How'd you do this week, Barb?" I said, glancing over at her and preparing to mark it on the chart. "I didn't weigh in," she finally replied. "Oh, well, the scale's empty now; you can go ahead." But Barbara made no move to go to the hall. Puzzled, I stopped what I was doing and looked at her. She looked like she was angry, but that couldn't—"Why do I have to weigh in, anyway?" She *was* angry. "Because," I answered calmly, too surprised at first to get angry myself, "it's a discipline every one of us in 3D agreed to." And for a split second, I wondered why *did* she have to weigh in? Why do any of these women with such nice figures have to bother weighing in? But something inside me checked that response before I could speak it.

Barbara still made no move to get up. I sensed that she might have picked up my slight hesitation, so I repeated my direction to her with some firmness in my voice. "Go on out now, Barb, and weigh in." "I don't think I should have to weigh in, if I don't want to." "Well, none of us particularly enjoys weighing in either, but that's the direction God has given us. So, be obedient."

She contemplated a further reply, then got up and stalked out to the scale in the hall. But the next thing I heard was her berating Dorcas, who was doing the weighing-in, about how stupid it was to have everyone weigh in! I shook my head, got up, and went out to the scale, speaking even before Dorcas could respond. "Barbara, your attitude is wrong!" I said, surprised at how strong the words came out. "I just spoke to you in the chapel about why everyone weighs in—because it's God's direction—and it is totally unnecessary for you to go on like this now with Dorcas."

Inside, I was wincing. Barbara worked in the church office, and I certainly didn't want to affect my relationship with her. But as much as I hated this confrontation, it was necessary to insist that she weigh in like everyone else. She weighed a perfect 110 pounds, according to her card, and I could not imagine for the life of me what she was reacting to.

She took her shoes off slowly, indicating she was going to get on the scale, so I returned to the chapel. Minutes passed, and another member came in from the hall, reported her weight loss, and sat down. Wait a minute, where was Barb? Had she left the building? Had I been too strong on her? I felt awful. Should I have excused her from weighing in? But had I done that. . . . A movement caught the corner of my eye. It was Barbara coming back, not to the seat she had occupied before, but to one closer to the outside door. "What was your weight loss, Barb?" I asked, trying to make it sound casual. "I gained—a pound and a half" she shot back, not raising her head to even look at me.

I marked her gain on the large, poster-type chart that had a place beside each name to mark the weight change for each week. And at the bottom was a place to total the group's combined weight loss for the week. Though everyone else in the group had a minus figure beside her name, none of us gave another thought to her gain—after all, even at 111½ she looked far better than most of the rest of us.

We prayed and started the meeting but had hardly begun, when I noticed that Barbara was crying. Lord, what do I do now? Then she spoke. "I—I'm really sorry for my weight gain. It affects the group's total," and then she began to sob. "Don't be silly, Barb! I wish I could gain one and a half pounds and look like you do!" one of the heavy group members said, trying to get her to smile.

But she cried inconsolably, her upset far surpassing the situation itself. Again she tried to talk. "I'm sorry. . . ." "Why are you so upset?" I asked. "It can't be over a measly pound and a half." "Everyone here lost weight tonight but me—that's awful!" And again she sobbed, burying her face in her hands.

Why had I ever made her weigh in? If only I had known—known what? Now my own emotions were getting involved, and I was losing my sense of any direction from God. I didn't want to see her so upset. Lord, help her! Lord, help me! The room was silent, and it felt as if everyone else was praying, too. "I never should have joined 3D!" Barbara burst out. "Dick and I had really begun to find something in this church that we had never known before. And, from what I had heard about it, I thought 3D would help me, but instead, I'm ruining the group!" "Now that is *not* true," Dorcas replied emphatically, "not true at all!" But there was a wall now between Barbara and the rest of the group, as if she had sealed herself off from us, brick by brick. She would not accept the assurance of the group, no matter what any of them said.

Then one of the women hit upon the thing that finally broke through the wall. "Are you afraid that the group will reject you because you are the only one that didn't lose weight?"

Startled, Barbara looked at the woman and nodded. Her thoughts were finally exposed, and it was okay. "I always worked hard at doing whatever the group I was in was doing. That way I knew I would be accepted. And if I couldn't, I'd drop out rather than fail." She went on and expressed her panic with this group. "Dieting has never been much of a problem with me. I've always been able to maintain my weight very close to what I've wanted it to be. But I've never been weighed in by anyone every single week like this. And to tell the truth, I've been a wreck every day just thinking about it. I find myself hopping on the scale twice a day at home, watching every quarter of a pound! Dick gets so upset with me. But I've seen how much every little quarter of a pound means to most of you, and how hard it is for you to lose each week. I didn't want to hurt the group!"

Now I was beginning to understand what all was going on inside of her. Because she was thin to begin with, she had felt perfectly acceptable in the group. It was as if she had passed some qualification for membership in her own mind. But any weight gain meant to her that she was failing both herself and the group. And she was irrationally scared to death the group would reject her. At this point, one of the heaviest women in the group spoke up and said a very beautiful thing to her. "I think there's something I ought to tell you. I've never felt accepted anywhere, because I'm so fat, and that includes church groups. I'm always sure I'll be rejected. I walk into a group, and I'm afraid no one will want to sit near me or talk to me, because I'm so fat!" She paused. "But now I see that you are just as afraid of rejection as I am, and the truth is that it doesn't have much to do with whether we are fat or thin. We are all scared of other peoples' opinions of us."

She went over and put her arm around Barbara, who cried freely, and then started laughing. "You know, I just can't believe this! I really can't believe it! I feel like someone just unlocked the door and let me go free."

Good grief! I was crying again, it was so beautiful; but then, so were most of the others. There was a fresh burst of laughter, as someone started the Kleenex box around the circle. And then others in the group confessed their fears of being rejected by the group, either because of their weight problems or their disorganized homes, or because they weren't as spiritually on top of things as they thought others might expect them to be. I was free to share my own fears of rejection and what a hold they had on me as I went into new situations.

It was clear that there wasn't a choice between any of us, fat or thin, leader or member. And all this had come to pass because one attractive, thin woman had gained a pound and a half. And to think that in the beginning I had regretted it coming up! God knew what He was doing, and it didn't matter if I didn't. After all, He was in charge, wasn't He? I needed to be willing to let people be uncomfortable, and be uncomfortable myself, to allow the Spirit of God to touch wherever He willed, using whatever method He chose. He took very good care of Barbara, and she was none the worse for all that crying; in fact, the whole thing had helped her *and* the group immeasurably, in spite of my ineptitude.

Similar situations occurred week after week in these three groups. And in each instance, we were in uncharted waters, praying much and leaning heavily on the Holy Spirit, for His wisdom and discernment. Much practical teaching was coming out of such seemingly petty experiences as thin people weighing in. But it certainly wasn't insignificant to realize, for instance, that you lived in constant fear of being rejected, or that you basically didn't trust other people, which several women discovered about themselves. That big hospital scale, which some of us called the "gray monster," was bringing up all sorts of opportunities for spiritual growth.

Another significant thing happened in the group that met upstairs on Tuesday evenings. The room itself was rather dismal—dirty gray walls, one funny-shaped window with a fan half blocking it, the worst of the church's folding chairs (most of them half broken, it seemed), and an ugly old beige rug on the floor. The fluorescent light fixture was broken, and the bare tubes were too bright and harsh for the smallness of the room. I remember Diane commenting that it felt as though we were in a police lineup room waiting to be interrogated, instead of a church diet group. But we did our best to forget the ugliness of the room and have good meetings in spite of it.

On this particular Tuesday night, Helen was talking. One of the original ten, Helen was a part of this new group, along with Ruth. As usual, Helen's whispery voice was hard to hear, especially if she was sharing something rather personal or difficult, which was the case this night. I can't remember what she was sharing, but she seemed to be talking into her lap in this barely audible voice, pausing after every three or four words. Before I knew what I was doing, strong words were coming out of my mouth. "Helen, *when are you going to grow up?*" The words shocked her, and me too. It was as if I'd had the thought out loud. I immediately tried to soften it. "I really think you need to stop talking and acting like a little girl and grow up into the woman of God you are supposed to be." The words were still strong, although not quite as loud.

Dorcas spoke up then, for which I was deeply grateful. The room had tensed up some, and it seemed as though a few in the group were embarrassed for Helen and perhaps upset with me. "I think Carol is absolutely right," Dorcas said. "I have been in groups with you for many months, and I have often felt that your soft, tender voice is very little-girlish. You are raising three teenage boys at home, aren't you? Is that the voice you use with them?" "Oh, no!" she quickly answered, with some volume in her voice. "I yell at John and the boys a lot at home." The group laughed at the quickness of her reply. "Then maybe you need to ask God why it is that here at church you come across so meek and mild, with a voice so timid it can't be heard," Dorcas went on.

Helen nodded her head but I wasn't sure she had understood at all what we were saying. She never spoke again for the rest of the meeting time.

I could hardly keep my mind on the rest of the group, worrying about whether I had done the right thing by confronting Helen so strongly right in the group. There was no question that there was an uncomfortable apprehension in the group after that. It had not been our style in the 3D groups to speak so strongly and directly to someone. I remained upset inside through the remainder of the meeting, and when the last woman walked out after the group, I closed the door, sinking fast. "What on earth ever made me speak so strongly to Helen?" I moaned to Dorcas. "I'll bet I've lost some friends tonight." "I think you were obeying the Holy Spirit. Helen *needed* it. What you were showing her was real love—tough love. I don't think she would have heard it at all if it had been said lovingly and softly."

And Dorcas went on to recall several small-group experiences where a whole group had spoken to Helen about talking up more. "Everyone had pointed it out—lovingly—but nothing has changed."

No matter what Dorcas said that night, I still felt totally wrong about what had happened. I was in self-pity up to my ears. Now I was the one who was refusing to listen to the truth.

When I got home, Bill immediately sensed my being "down." I told him what had happened, and he spoke to me even more strongly than Dorcas. "God has placed you in a position of leadership in that group, not because you wanted to be a leader, but because God put you there. And if His Holy Spirit is going to help you lead His way, you have to be willing to say what your heart tells you is necessary, regardless of how it comes across." He paused. "And if you refuse to speak because you are afraid someone might not want to hear it or like it, you are wrong!"

And I saw that I didn't care as much about Helen and how she was taking what I had said, as I was caring about me.

"I think you said exactly what God gave you to say," he went on, "and what's more, I think it needed to be said strongly. Your trouble is, you're really more concerned about people liking you than helping someone like Helen grow in Christ."

I clammed up. I was not about to discuss my old fear of rejection again. I just wanted to forget that whole episode. It was pointless to talk about it further. He would see! Next Tuesday night, the only people who would show up for the group would be Dorcas and me.

The first thing the next morning, Dorcas called me and said Helen had called, crying, and wanted to talk to both of us. I knew it! What a mess I'd made!

But as it turned out, it was not a mess at all. Helen shared lots and lots of things that she needed to share. God had really used that confrontation to open up areas of her life that needed healing. I was awed at what God did in her life that day and throughout the rest of the week. We met with her, then Bill met with her, and most important, God met with her, in a new and exciting way, and she practically "grew up" right before our eyes.

The next Tuesday night Helen was in the best shape ever. She could hardly wait to tell how God had spoken to her and healed her of many fears and hurts. Like so many of the rest of us, she feared rejection. "I guess I've had an image of a good Christian—it was someone who never spoke loudly or raised her voice."

No wonder she had looked so blankly at me that night. I had jumped out of the "good Christian" box by speaking so strongly and loudly. "And at home," Helen smiled, "where I have to raise my voice so frequently, I felt like a total failure as a Christian. So I tried to be someone else at church, and everyone likes little girls, so that seemed like a safe place to hide." "What I really want," she said, drawing herself up straight in her chair and looking at each woman in the circle, "is to be myself." Her voice was strong and clear now. "And with God's help, I'm going to be." We practically cheered. She was so much freer than we had ever seen her. "And I want you all to tell me," she concluded, "whenever I sink back into that little-girl syndrome." We all laughed and promised to tell her.

Jan spoke up after that. "I can't tell you what a help it was to me last week to learn that Helen raised her voice at home and even yelled at her boys. I've been living in such self-condemnation, because now that I've become the instant mother of two teenage sons"— she had just married a widower in the church—"I'm always yelling at home, and I guess I, too, believed that good Christian mothers just didn't do that. I had felt so defeated in my Christian life—until last week. For the first time, I didn't feel all alone."

Others agreed with what Jan was saying. Practically everyone had gotten some sort of blessing out of it, however unexpected. God had used the confrontation with Helen to speak to each of us. I silently asked Him to forgive me for having wanted to avoid what He had intended to use, just as I had before with Barbara in the other group.

ℒ

It hardly seemed possible that the three months of these second 3D groups were just about over! We decided to conclude by having a potluck dinner with all three groups together on the last Tuesday night. But as we were making plans and deciding what to ask everyone to bring, we felt a check from the Lord. We listened, knowing that God was trying to get our attention about something. And what we felt was that we, the leaders, were to plan, cook, and serve the meal. The dinner menu was to be a surprise for the 3Ders, and the whole occasion was to be an evening out for them. They loved the idea when we shared it with them. "Dress up, and come prepared to celebrate," we announced. "We'll have a special last night together."

And again, without our realizing it, God was leading us through this celebration into a deeper awareness of a very important aspect of 3D: that the leaders were there for one purpose—to serve.

April 2 arrived, and it was a beautiful evening. The aroma of roasting beef filled the church, and it was the first thing we noticed the moment we opened the door. Ruth had shopped at the farmers' market for fresh vegetables and was readying platters of broccoli, cauliflower, and carrots. Potatoes were baked, then mashed and stuffed back in the shells with a little bit of grated cheese sprinkled on them. And for dessert we were having chilled cups of fresh fruit—diced apples, mixed with sliced peaches, fresh strawberries, and blueberries, and cantaloupe balls. We arranged it carefully so that it all looked as good as it smelled. A children's Sunday school classroom was somehow given the atmosphere of a private dining room, with crisp white tablecloths and centerpieces of candles surrounded by arrangements of fresh-cut flowers, and other touches that came to us as we worked.

The women could hardly believe their eyes when they walked in! We suggested that they seat themselves next to someone from one of the other groups, rather than someone from their own group. There was no hesitation, and within minutes the room was filled with laughter and animated conversation.

We had invited Fred, an elder of the church and a good soloist, to help us with some special music. He did a fine job, and we were drawn together in song and then in sharing. The evening couldn't have been nicer, and the groups had a surprise for Dorcas and me. They presented us with lovely watches, which, they told us, were symbolic of the time we had given them. We were deeply moved. The love of God permeated that evening from the beginning to the end.

What more could He do, I wondered. He had certainly blessed us in and through the 3D groups, even though we had never had any idea of where He was leading us. At this point, almost everyone in the three groups wanted to continue in 3D. And we decided that we would—but how it was going to work, or what we were going to do next, only God knew.

TEN

LEARNING TO RECEIVE

Outside the new social hall, I glanced at the coat rack and had to smile. There were hardly any coats there, even though it was still April and not what anyone would call a warm spring evening. Being a long-time dieter myself, I knew only too well the significance of shedding winter coats. The illusion that overweight people have—that a coat can hide twenty or twenty-five pounds—works the other way, as well. The successful dieter can't wait to get her winter coat put away. She'll take it off, usually too soon, and will shiver a little, if necessary, to show off her new figure.

Tonight was another orientation meeting, and again we had asked those 3Ders who wanted to continue, to come early. Most of them had lost a great deal of weight—hence the empty coat racks. Shivering a little myself, I went inside. There were thirty-four veteran 3Ders sitting in the rows, excited and eager to begin again. And by eight o'clock some thirty or so new women, a number of them with their coats still on, had come to hear about the program and ask questions. "I can't believe this; I really can't believe it!" I kept saying to myself, and then remembered that I'd said the same thing three months before, at the beginning of 1974. "What is God doing? "I whispered to Dorcas. "I haven't the vaguest idea," she replied, with a shrug, "but I guess we'd better get started."

We walked to the front of the room. I took a deep breath and said, "If we look shocked and surprised—and scared—it's because we are!" And from there, we let the Holy Spirit lead us in what to share, letting them know exactly what they were getting into, and how much it was going to involve in terms of time and commitment. When everything we could think of was covered, several women who had completed their first three months spoke up.

Mary was the first to stand up, and I was surprised, because she had remained relatively quiet during most of the weeks the group had met. Nor had we felt any leading in that group to draw Mary out. She had cried almost every week, not that noticeably, but tears were falling continually. We sensed that those tears had something to do with the accidental death of her youngest son several months before, but we clearly felt the Holy Spirit saying, "Just let her cry. Those are tears of healing." And so we did. Tonight, apparently, she had decided to speak. The tears came again, before she could get the first words out, and then, "Most of you know that Tom and I lost our son Jim last October, very suddenly. . . ." She cried some more, and someone handed her the Kleenex box. (We had learned to always have a box of Kleenex nearby.)

The room was perfectly still; you could feel people praying for Mary. It was extremely difficult for her to say what she wanted and needed to say, but she was determined to keep going. "It was an awful shock to us, but we did our best to accept it. We felt that, after all, God had allowed it to happen, and as Christians we were supposed to accept it and go on. Well, that sounds good, but the way I wound up handling my hurt was to eat every time I felt any grief, and in those first months, that was most of the time. In four months I had gained twenty-five pounds." She had regained her composure now and went on much more easily. "We had joined Parkminster only a few days before Jim died. Everyone was wonderful to us—friends at church and our family—and we wanted so much to have it all together for them. So we put on a victorious attitude when we went out, but in the privacy of our home we were crying lots."

I hurt, in my heart, as I listened to Mary. Many times I had been concerned about how she and Tom were doing, but each time I had seen them, they seemed so good that I had backed away from asking. I didn't want to bring up any unnecessary hurt by mentioning the whole thing. But now, listening to her, I realized how selfish I had been. I had chosen to believe what I had seen on the outside, and had not wanted to make even a suggestion that might have given them the opportunity to express the grief they were keeping bottled up. "I joined 3D," Mary went on, "because I wanted to lose that weight, and I did. But that was only a small part of what happened to me. In 3D, I found that not only was it okay to cry in public, it was okay to hurt as a Christian, and it was okay to express that hurt to Christians. And once I was free to express some of that hurt, just by crying in my group, I began to experience God's healing deep inside." She smiled and said, "The twenty-five pounds were nothing more than stored-up tears that finally had a chance to come out." She hesitated. "You will never know," and here she sought the eyes of the others who had been in her group, "how much I appreciated your love and understanding, even though you never actually spoke to me about it. I think I know Jesus better now because of you."

She sat down with a big smile, and her eyes were sparkling. But there was hardly a dry eye in the room. Wiping the tears from my own eyes, I said, "Well, Mary, if shedding tears will take the pounds off, a lot of us are going to go home thinner tonight."

Testimony followed testimony after that—they were just popping up all over the room. And finally I had to step in and stop them, so we could get on with the meeting. The result of the evening was that sixty women signed up for 3D groups.

At the rate 3D was growing, all kinds of decisions were now necessary, and Bill suggested that we quickly get ourselves under the direction of the Session (the ruling board of a local Presbyterian church). And we did. By June 1974 there were six 3D groups going simultaneously, and I was beginning to eat, sleep, and even dream 3D, to the exclusion of all else—the dangerous exclusion of all else, though I didn't see that at the time.

ر

Summer brought with it an opportunity for a complete change of pace, and I was delighted. Our new cottage on Cape Cod had been under construction since April and was at last nearing completion. We had decided to take three weeks of our August vacation a month early, in order to be able to work around the place and do some of the necessary jobs to make the cottage livable. And so, not long after the children finished school, we packed up and were off to Cape Cod. But what we had thought would be small finishing touches, like painting and varnishing, turned out to be considerably more than that. All the windows, inside and out, had to be either stained or painted—on both the first and second floors! We wanted the inside woodwork to remain natural, so three coats of polyurethane needed to be applied. And then there was the floor tile in the front hall, and the wallpapering we wanted in the kitchen and bathroom, and putting in a front lawn—if we had time. By the end of the three weeks we were less than half finished! Bill and I decided that the children and I should stay on for the remainder of the summer, and he would join us at the end of August.

I did little or no thinking about 3D during those busy summer months. In fact, the only time it came to mind was when a steady procession of visitors from Rochester kept appearing at the front door to visit and help. It was an unbelievable experience. Day after day, I would look out the window and see friends from church stopping out front. They knew I was there alone with the children and could use all the help I could get. We had room for the first few, but others camped down the road, and still others were staying at motels nearby. And in just about every case, it was a 3Der and her family.

Something else had happened during those nine months we had 3D groups. There was now a feeling of family and friends between us, instead of minister and parishioners. I loved having them drop in, and they got so much of the work done that there was little left for Bill to finish in August, and he was actually able to come and just relax for the last week of his vacation rather than work frantically to finish by Labor Day. But inevitably, with ten or twelve people living in an unfinished house with one bathroom, mixed in with the blessings were bound to be some times when our 3D experience of being open and honest with one another came in handy. There was, for instance, the time when Marilyn, the petite 3Der who had once been concerned about praying for forty women, arrived with her husband Bill and their four children—twin boys age fourteen, a girl age thirteen, and another, age ten. It happened that they were the church's wallpapering experts, and they heard we needed help to paper two rooms. They did a terrific job of wallpapering and put a lot of time into it, and I was very grateful. When the time came for them to begin their long trip home, I started making all sorts of plans for lunches for their trip, including baking some cookies and making fudge brownies and mixing up lots of lemonade. "Oh, Carol, please don't," Marilyn said. "We were really looking forward to stopping on the way home." "But," I insisted, "it will save lots of time and money to have a lunch with you." She was very insistent I not do it, but I was determined that I was going to do it, no matter what she said.

Finally, Marilyn raised her voice, and it was shaking. "Why can't you just once be on the receiving end! You do so much for all of us back at church, and for a change we have a chance to do something for you. But you won't let us!" She got up and walked out of the room, and so caught up was I in doing what I had planned on, that I still was unaware of how deeply she meant what she was saying. I continued setting out the necessary things to make the lunches. When she came back in and saw me, she burst out crying. "You didn't even listen to me, did you? We came, because we felt God wanted *us* to help *you!*"

It seemed to me she was making a very big deal out of nothing, but at last I stopped, to try to hear what she was saying. "Why won't you just let us help you and stop insisting on outdoing us and giving back every way you can? We need to give, and you need to know how to receive." Suddenly, finally, I heard God speaking to me. And the only reason I could finally begin to hear Him was that Marilyn had been willing to make a scene. Her honesty penetrated my massive insensitivity—of doing the "right thing" because it made me feel good.

All at once, I saw it and was stunned. I asked Marilyn to forgive me. Later, munching on one of the sandwiches I had made for them, I saw still more about why I was so compulsive about doing for others— indeed, why I was happiest when I was busy doing, doing, doing. It was another deeper level of my drive for acceptance. If I did enough for them, "they" (whoever "they" happened to be) would have to accept me. As I thought about that, I somehow saw that my life-long scramble to do for others in order to be accepted was going to have to stop. Now, I could start doing for others simply because God gave me the nudge to do so, and it would be for His glory and not mine.

ELEVEN

IN LEADING, THEY WERE LED

"September 25th, 1974, 8:00 PM" the announcement had read, and by eight, there were more than 150 women gathered at the church for our third orientation meeting. Word about 3D had spread all over the city, and women from many churches were there to hear about the new Christian diet program. And when we had finished laying it on the line—and we made very sure that no one was entering under any false conceptions—127 of them signed up.

The most immediate problem we faced was leadership. Figuring each team of leaders could lead two groups, that still meant we were going to need a dozen leaders. Where were we going to find them? After a lot of emergency praying, the solution we came up with was to approach those old 3D hands, whom God seemed to be saying were ready to assume the responsibility of group leadership. Almost to a woman, they protested, "Not me!" "But I still have so much to learn myself," Lois exclaimed. "And I have more weight to lose," moaned Helen in her new clear voice. "I know, I know," I replied. "I felt exactly the same way when I was asked to lead the first group. I wanted to be in a 3D group so I could get help, but God called me to assume the responsibility of leading the group instead." I smiled. "I got more help than I expected—and not the way I thought it would come."

We talked a great deal about what a leader was supposed to be and what qualifications she should have. And we were reminded of the leaders whom God had called out from the beginning of time—weak and needy individuals, whose hearts were towards God and who loved Him. They were not persons of brilliance of mind or eloquent speech—Moses had a stuttering problem—but they were believers who were committed to serving God in any way that He called them to. "The essential qualification for leading people is still the same," I said, smiling, "and that's a commitment to God and a willingness to serve Him wherever you are called. Are you willing?"

And so twelve old-timers took their places as 3D leaders, scared but willing to step out on faith. They were delighted that they could work in teams of two, rather than alone, and that made the call a good deal easier to accept. But, since the details of the program were still evolving week by week before our eyes, and we had no manual or instructions about how to conduct a successful 3D session, they were sent into groups dependent totally on God's guidance.

Dorcas and I continued to lead several groups, but increasingly we saw more clearly that our own call was evolving, too—to work more with the leaders themselves. They needed direction, encouragement, and counsel from us. And as we met with them weekly, we found our times of sharing together an invaluable experience. We were all growing in our relationship with the Lord because He was demanding more from us than any of us felt equipped to handle. We didn't know how to lead leaders, and the leaders didn't know how to lead groups. So together we sought more of the wisdom and direction of God—watching as before our eyes, lives were being changed.

God was at work in all of us, and we knew it. We also began to come into some sense of the meaning of a "call" being for lay people, as well as for ministers and missionaries. "You did not choose me, but I have chosen you . . ." (John 15:16) was a verse most of us thought belonged to the full-time Christian worker only. Now we saw it was for us, too.

God's sense of humor also became apparent to all of us, as we worked together over those next three months. It was uncanny how often the leaders would have in their particular group, not just one, but two or more persons with exactly the same problems they had. Thus, through their speaking up in the group to someone else, God spoke directly to their own hearts. Ruth found that she had a number of women who wanted to escape responsibilities and slip off to bed or to read a good "Christian" book. She had to speak strongly to them about being obedient to God, and in a couple of cases, she and her partner even helped them to get on a daily time schedule. She was able to speak with authority from her own experience, which now had become a tremendous asset. And each time, God turned the words right around and grounded them even deeper into her own life.

The same was true of Lois and Marilyn, who were both quiet in outward personality and who had several women in their group who simply refused to share of themselves. They saw how difficult it was for a group when one or two people would steadfastly refuse to open up. And again, by encouraging others to share, they became even freer themselves.

God was working uniquely in the leaders, in a way most of them had not experienced before—in leading, they were being led.

Behind the scenes of 3D, God was giving Bill very definite teachings to be used in the groups, as well as key Scripture memory verses. We also were seeing the outlines for the members' disciplines. As each unfolded, we would type it up as fast as we could, run copies off, and pass them out in groups for weekly use. It was phenomenal, and we knew it was God, because the content was coming too quickly for it to be us. We made up Scripture verse cards to take home, found books and pamphlets to read, tapes to listen to, and even bought a second "gray monster" scale.

And for our expenses, we were now collecting a dollar per member per week. Someone was convicted that we needed to be disciplined in our finances as well as our food, and we knew that was the word of God to us. With these funds we bought tape recorders for group use, and Bill was then able to put the weekly teachings on tape, eliminating his need to be in every group.

Still the 3D program kept growing—nearly doubling in size, every time we opened it for new members. By spring 1975 there were twenty-two groups meeting at Parkminster, and in addition, we had well over thirty leaders, necessitating several leaders' groups besides. A Free Methodist church in the community and also a Roman Catholic church were now asking if they could begin groups with our help, an offer for which we were grateful, because every square inch of space at the church was being taken up by 3D groups, and we were having to turn people away.

Indeed, God was working in such a supernatural way through the expansion and growth of the 3D program, that I should have been watching a little more closely for the enemy of God to come sneaking up from behind. I had had more than one warning that things were getting out of kilter, but I had not listened. While I was on a retreat at the Community of Jesus, several people had remarked how much my life seemed to be wrapped up in 3D. Well, I thought to myself, of course it is. After all, there are over three hundred people involved in the program, and I am the one who bears the responsibility. They just didn't understand the demands and pressures that went along with running such a successful program.

Then, after the retreat was over, I sat down to talk with several of the women of the Community, who were direct and totally honest with me. "Frankly, Carol, you come on more like a career woman than a mother," one of them said. "And you seem unaware that your children need you to listen to them, just as much as the women in 3D." She went on to tell me that she had happened to notice Betsy, our eight-year-old daughter, approach me during afternoon coffee hour the day before, very excitedly telling me about two twin sisters who were soon to arrive for a visit. "I don't think you even heard what she said, because your mind was on something else, and Betsy just wandered away, disappointed."

She was right. That was an exact replay of what had been happening at home all the time lately. The only thing on my mind for months had been 3D. I could not remember one significant thing that had happened for weeks to us as a family. It was devastating to me to realize this, and I broke down crying. I didn't have the slightest idea how I could get off this merry-go-round, but I wanted to.

Another woman from the Community spoke up and said that it wasn't the amount of time I was putting in on 3D; it was the attitude of my heart that was wrong. I wasn't sure what she meant by that, but I listened.

They were very loving to me, and at the same time very honest. Yes, their words stung—like Mercurochrome on a cut. But that stinging meant that the possibility of subsequent infection, which would hurt far, far more, was being arrested. But typically, I wanted an instant solution. "What can I do? I'm overwhelmed with the responsibilities of 3D and my family. There just aren't enough hours in the day." "Ask the Lord to help you," they said. "You are taking this 3D thing too much to yourself and not allowing God to carry the burdens and responsibilities."

I walked away from that discussion, feeling as I had when Cay and Judy had talked to me about my being so critical. I didn't know how I was going to change, but three months afterwards, I knew I was less critical. And remembering that word of truth reminded me of when Marilyn had told me how incapable I was of receiving from other people. In less than a year, I had learned more about myself and how I came across to others than I had learned over the previous twenty years.

Although I felt somewhat overwhelmed after this last confrontation, I knew it was absolutely right. So I began to try to forget 3D when I was home with the family. It helped, but I also sensed that while I was working hard to change my outside behavior again, there was more work necessary underneath. That, I had to leave to God. I couldn't change inside—that was His job. It would take time; I would have liked to sit around and just wait until I was all perfect, but 3D and my family kept moving rapidly around me. So I asked God to make me more aware of the needs of my family, and I made an attempt at caring more for them at home and listening, especially to the children.

By May 1975, 3D was blossoming in many of the churches around the area. A brief appearance on a nationally syndicated television talk show had deluged us with more than fifteen hundred letters of inquiry. Now we were known far beyond the immediate Rochester area, and all kinds of suggestions as to how to run the program better and what to do differently poured into the church office. Telephone calls were received from several different states, and people wanted help and counsel over the telephone and via the mail. It was incredible how many people, Christian people, were searching for help in these three areas of their lives—diet, discipline and discipleship.

The elders of the church decided to legally incorporate the program, appointing executive officers and a board of directors. "It is important that we follow and protect the direction in which God has been leading us," an elder said, "and not be tossed hither and yon by all these new suggestions."

He was right. We believed that God had been guiding us from the very beginning, and we did not want to lose the foundations He had laid. Some of the outside groups wanted more emphasis on the diet phase of the program, while others wanted to leave out the dieting and stress the spiritual disciplines more. And still others felt uncomfortable about any personal sharing or speaking truth in the groups, so they wanted this de-emphasized. It was sometimes hard to hear God amidst all these opinions.

In the meantime, as mute testimony to the effectiveness of the 3D program, with its strong emphasis on commitment, caring, openness, and honesty, we were seeing more and more lives being rapidly and beautifully altered. We were also beginning to see the profound connection between the basic attitudes of members and their eating habits. All kinds and degrees of rebellion, fear, and anxiety were surfacing in the groups.

Bubbling up everywhere were attitudes of self-pity among people who found it difficult to lose weight, and self-righteousness on the part of those who lost easily. We were indeed becoming the people God intended us to be—real, honest, and in need of a Savior to free us from ourselves.

We were also learning how to bring our poor attitudes into the light of God, there to confess them and to be forgiven so that we could move on. And to our utter astonishment, we lost a ton of weight in twelve weeks!

TWELVE

STEPPING OUT

"Carol, 3D is no longer God's answer to you; it has now become your answer to the hundreds of people involved in it." Judy Sorensen stopped and looked straight at me. "You're in danger of becoming a disciple of the 3D program, rather than a disciple of Jesus Christ."

Her words shook me. I had been making a real effort to care more for my family, and I had tried to unwrap myself as much as possible, whenever possible, from the demands of 3D, when they interfered with our home life. But Judy saw my problem differently. It was not something that I could just patch up with a few adjustments. She and Cay Andersen were in Rochester again, for another spring teaching mission at the church. It was May 1975. And while they were delighted to see that the 3D program had grown so large so quickly, and that God was using it all over the area, they were concerned about where I was spiritually. All week, during the mission, they had seen me running around, directing 3D leaders, hurrying in and out of groups, and so on.

Cay joined the conversation. "Whenever God is doing a work in the hearts and lives of people, be on guard for the big self moving into God's place. Only

God is allowed at the center of His work." She continued: "So, Carol, step out."

"Step out? You mean step out of 3D?" I asked in a barely audible voice. "Oh, no," she chuckled, "just out of God's place at the center." She made it sound so easy. In fact, to graphically demonstrate what she meant, she actually took a big step to the right of where she had been standing in Bill's office. "Just like this, out of the way, so God can get back in where He belongs." She laughed, but I couldn't; I wanted to quit the whole thing. I had been trying so hard since the women at the Community had spoken to me about my career-woman attitude. And evidently, it hadn't done a bit of good.

"Don't be so discouraged with yourself," she went on. "That's our sin nature, to move in on God's territory, and it's a continuing battle."

It seemed like a losing battle to me. But even in the midst of their strong warning to me, I saw the love of God again. This whole journey with my weight and my need for various disciplines was so that Jesus Christ might be glorified by my life. And I had slipped off course again. I had confused God's work with God Himself. I knew in my heart that I had lost a great deal of closeness to Him, and I knew it was because I was so caught up in all the nuts-and-bolts details of the organizational needs of 3D. I wasn't peaceful. And I had no joy. It was work, work, work.

And so, on that May afternoon, Cay and Judy spoke the words that God wanted me to hear. I couldn't keep from crying. The words had pierced my heart and soul. "How do I get out of the center of it?" I asked through my tears. "By an act of your will and with the help of God," Judy answered. "That's where it has to begin."

As they spoke further to me, the picture became clearer and clearer. I had closed out the rest of the life

"Tears of self-pity will only take you down into depression, while tears of repentance will take you out into life and joy."

Bill had been sitting very quietly beside me, not saying a word. But when I made no move to leave, he got up and opened the door of his office and said sternly, "Be obedient, Carol. The chapel's free and we'll see you in a while." I really wanted him to go with me. The last thing I wanted was to be alone now. I had no idea why, until I closed the door behind me in the chapel and knelt at the altar. Then it came to me. It had been so long since I had come to God alone and in need, that I had forgotten how to be in need and helpless before a Holy God. I had been using God every day to help me to be strong and have the wisdom and understanding to guide those entrusted to my care. I had been praying faithfully for my family and all thirty leaders, but I had forgotten much about my daily need of a Savior to save me from myself.

Sobbing as I knelt at that little altar, looking straight at the shiny gold cross, I saw my tear-stained face in it. It was a tired, hurt, strained face. I cried, "God, come close to me. I need you so much." But He seemed far from me.

I don't know how long I knelt and cried that afternoon, but it was an experience I'll never forget. Slowly, ever so slowly, as I looked at the cross, the reflection of my face disappeared. At first, it had been like a mirror instead of a cross. All I could see was me. Then the cross became more evident to me in its wholeness. And I began to feel the unexplainable presence of God. And the pain and hurt and disappointment began to lift. I knew it was going to be okay. God was now again moving into the center of my It felt good.

at church. There was no time to go to Bible study or circle meetings. With all those 3D groups meeting each week in the church, plus several in other churches in the community, and then the leadership responsibility for thirty leaders at Parkminster and ten or twelve others at Holy Ghost Church—there was no time, no time for anything but 3D! I didn't ask Bill much about anything else in the church. But instead, every time I got him to myself, I would pour a million questions on him—about 3D. Oh yes, I did shut it off, as best I could, at home with the children, but the minute they were out of my sight, I was chin deep in it again.

Suddenly, the smile face popped into my mind. Only now the words beneath it read differently: "Smile, Carol has the answer!" I felt sick. "How could I?" I moaned, and I made myself tell them what had just come into my mind. "What did you expect from a sinner?" Cay laughed again, and her laugh was warm and contagious.

I knew she wasn't making light of what I was seeing, but she was trying to help me get into reality and not go down in anguish and depression about my sudden realization. "Just go off by yourself," Judy suggested, "and give the whole program back to God and take your rightful position under Him."

I just wanted to sit there and cry. And again I had the feeling that in ten or fifteen minutes they had taken care of something that I thought would require at least a couple of hours. "There's no one in the chapel now, so why don't you go down by yourself and talk it out with the Lord. And you can cry all you want! Only be sure those are tears of repentance and not self-pity," Judy cautioned.

Someone had once told me the difference between those two kinds of tears, and I had never forgot it.

It was through that experience that the third D of the 3D program took on a much greater significance to me. God had personally walked me through the defeat and discouragement of a weight problem into some semblance of victory, so that I could share with others. Then He had been teaching me a great deal about the amazing freedom that comes through discipline. And now I had touched on the very core of it all—what it really meant to be a disciple of Jesus Christ.

I had deceived myself into thinking that because it was Christian work that I was so deeply involved in, God was automatically at the center. It was a mistake I had made over and over again in my Christian life. But many of the things I had done in the name of Christ, I now saw were centered on me, not Him. And God blessed them anyway, in spite of me. But now He was beginning to show me what it meant to be His disciple.

Things were different after that. I finally understood what the Community women had meant when they told me, "It isn't the amount of time you are giving to 3D; it's your heart attitude that is wrong."

I had to laugh; it was so simple. There was room for only one of us, Him or me, at the center of 3D, and as long as I was occupying that place, He was not about to. As much as my ego might have wanted to remain there, I really wanted Him there, not me. And so, by His grace and mercy, I was able to take that giant step that Cay Andersen had talked about. And, funny thing: When I stepped out of the center, I found I was stepping into Christ.

THIRTEEN

MOVING ON

In the back of our garage there was a small, one-person office. In the center of the uncluttered desk lay a memo from Lillian, my publisher. Paraclete Press was about to reissue the ongoing bestseller *3D,* which I'd written 24 years before. She was asking me to revise it where needed, and to provide a new conclusion, letting the reader know what had happened to 3D (and me) in the interim.

The deadline was the end of August. With time growing daily shorter, my false starts grew increasingly desperate and my prayers more earnest.

I had written over 20,000 words about the ups and downs of the 3D program, and had talked about the growth and outreach of the program since 1975. The time line, complete with facts and figures from then until now, was impressive and was a wonderful writing exercise. But the truth was, it wouldn't edify or encourage anyone in need who picked up this book.

My daily prayer journal was full of questions to the Lord: "What do you want me to say? Do you want me to share this particular fact or this event?" There was a lot of ground to cover in both 3D and in my own life in order to bring the book up to date and to a new conclusion. And lying just beneath the surface was the fact that I still had to battle my weight. I wondered if knowing this would be a disappointment to the reader of the book.

"Lord, how can I revise the *3D* book when I still struggle with my weight so much?"—I often asked that question of the Lord in my quiet time. I was encouraged when I read, in the front of my journal, that Teresa of Avila had recommended that her sisters write whatever God was saying to them "interiorly."

These were the words that seemed to come to my heart:

> *It isn't your weight that has any ability or disability to glorify me. It is you, my child. You, wrapped up with my love and my wonder. You, the recipient of my mercy, my compassion, and my understanding. I do not think the way you think. Your talk about weight is foreign to me. Do you really believe all thin people glorify me? You know better. No, no, my child, you are missing the picture. My will is all you need to be concerned about. And you have to discern that daily for your life. So write about my love and my mercy, my compassion and my understanding.*

❧

"Please, Lord, let David be satisfied," I thought, as I sat in my editor's office.

"The reason the *3D* book has touched so many lives, Carol," David reminded me as he went over the pages I had brought him, "is that you were willing to be very needy and vulnerable. And people could identify with you and could fit right into your shoes with their own needs."

"This is good," he finally said. "But it's more theme-oriented than life-centered."

"I hear you, David." Even more important, I could hear the Lord speaking to me through David's words.

"Sit and listen," David added as I left his office. "God will speak to you and show you exactly what to write."

"Well," I thought to myself, "He did speak to me in my quiet time, about mercy and love and compassion."

David was confident in God. But I was scared.

I did pray. And I kept writing in my prayer journal. But my prayers sounded more like plea-bargaining than real prayer. I still wasn't making the clear connection between my prayers and my writing. Too often I would quit praying and go to the computer to write. I wasn't getting it. And to my repeated dismay, what came out was just words on a page, without even a dull sparkle.

"3D opened groups on twelve military airbases—three in Alaska, three in Germany, two in Hawaii, one in New Jersey, two in California, and one in Texas."

"3D conferences in Rochester outgrew the church facilities and moved downtown to a large hotel to host over 500 participants from around the country."

"Television, radio, and speaking engagements tripled in 1980."

Boring! How will this information increase the faith of the reader?

More prayer, more typing. The same response from my editor: "Good, but not there yet. Remember, the number one enemy of best is good."

"Lord, open up my life and my heart on these pages," I prayed, "so that again I may connect with the reader and share what you have done and are doing in the program and in my own life."

Watch out when you pray prayers like that! God does take you at your word. Vulnerability—the painful kind—was just around the corner for me.

❧

On July 17, two weeks into the project, at four o'clock in the morning, my pet of 14 years, Joshua—a Manchester toy terrier—became desperately sick. I did all I could to make him comfortable, but nothing helped. I was going to have to face one of the most difficult decisions a pet owner has to face. Was it time to put him to sleep?

Circumstances had forced my hand: Joshua was old and ill. Suffering with degenerating back disc problems, he could no longer walk without falling over. And now, not only were his back legs swelling, so was his right front leg. And finally he was sick—uncontrollably sick—in the middle of the night.

My only thoughts were of my companion and what I could do for him. But I realized that by putting off my own pain regarding this decision, I was keeping him in pain. Still, I wasn't ready. I thought that surely I had another six months, even though my vet, Dr. Hickey, was now giving him cortisone shots to alleviate his pain.

I had been praying about it, trusting that God would show me the right time. But not yet. Not now. Despite my protests, my heart knew *this* was the day. There's no point going into detail; anyone who's lost a beloved pet does not need to revisit that sorrow. At the end of the day Joshua was dead and I was devastated.

The event crossed my will and my emotions far more deeply than I expected. I kept waiting for time to heal the wound, but it didn't. The next day was as raw as the first. I forced myself to go back out to the garage to try to work on the *3D* project, but invariably my eyes filled with tears, and for the next 15 minutes I would cry.

For 14 years Joshua had slept at the bottom of our bed. Manchesters are often one-person dogs, preferring to sleep as close to their master's pillow as possible. Bill and I had a good marriage (40 years this past October), but Joshua on my pillow didn't fly. Joshua didn't mind; the bottom of the bed with his blanket and my feet was the best spot in the world, as far as he was concerned.

But now he was gone.

Not everyone liked Joshua—he barked a lot and did his job well of protecting the house and me. UPS always left our packages on the front steps instead of knocking on the door. From the sound of the barking inside, one would have thought we had a Doberman Pinscher behind the door, instead of a miniature terrier. But he was soft as a teddy bear with me—and that made the break even tougher.

My feelings frustrated me—they were too much on the surface, and they were getting in the way of my job, I thought.

I kept crying and I kept trying to write. I didn't have to pretend I wasn't hurting. This was real, this was me, and I could cry. It didn't matter what people thought. And every day God talked to me about deep things in my soul. He was healing deep pockets of grief. My mother died quite young, my father died suddenly— and more recently my brother died abruptly. I had handled all those griefs the best way I knew how. But now we were going deeper.

One rainy afternoon, nine days after Joshua's death, I was sitting at the desk. The latest page was up on the computer's monitor, but I was not looking at it. I was staring out the window. Rain was lashing the window, blurring my view of the backyard. But I could still see the tiny pine sapling planted between two big pines. The tall trees reached out their low branches and joined them above the little one—protecting it, making it almost like a grotto. The small white pottery vase filled with green-and-white variegated ivy and yellow sunflowers was still standing, but the one with pink and white lilies had fallen over.

Our daughter, Liz, had brought the pine sapling to me the day Joshua died. And we planted it to remind us of Joshua. It was a miniature pine, just as he was a miniature terrier.

Without warning, like a wave of the sea, grief rolled over me, starting in the pit of my stomach and creeping up to that secret hiding place for tears. They slipped out one at a time. "I miss you, Joshua," I whispered, "I miss you so much."

I forced myself to turn back to the project. There was a knock on the door, and in walked my friend Mary, a sales representative for Paraclete Press. She was checking up on me, since over a week had passed since Joshua died. "How are you doing, my friend?" she asked.

"Well, Mary, if the truth be known, I just had another good cry for myself." She wasn't surprised.

Then Mary told me of an experience she'd had a few weeks before. She was talking to a counselor who had purchased several videos and prayer books on grief. Discussing the needs of grieving people, Mary asked him about his therapy groups: How big were the groups? Were people able to express their grief with strangers? Were there more women than men? Were their grief situations similar?

"In a typical group there are parents working through the suicide of their son, two people grieving over recent divorces, a mother with a runaway daughter, a man whose mother just died—and two people who lost pets."

"Pets?"

"Grief is grief," he told Mary. "When people express their feelings, you begin to understand that grief has no boundaries. It feels the same, though the circumstances are different." He paused. "I wasn't sure, the first time I let a woman in who'd lost her dog, how the others would feel. I was pleasantly surprised. She received full support and acceptance. And once word got out that I'd accept people grieving over the loss of a pet, I've hardly had a group without at least one person there because of a pet."

I smiled. "Thanks, Mary. I needed to hear that."

I could stop feeling so stupid about the depth of my feelings about Joshua.

❧

This conversation made me think a lot about diet, and particularly 3D.

Weight control, whether a person is overweight or too thin, only starts the process of help. Hidden beneath this all-consuming problem lies much more that needs the love and mercy and compassion of God. But we start with the outside. It's safer. We can test the water and see if there is love and understanding for us with a personal need. We have a problem with weight, and our need is already obvious. So we might just as well talk about it.

More often than not, the "stuff" inside doesn't help the weight problem on the outside. Though not directly connected, they seem to feed off each other. Like the chicken or the egg, it is impossible to say which came first. Did one gain weight because one had a low self-image or was full of self-pity and anger? Or did gaining weight create and magnify those already existing problems?

My mind turned back to those 3D beginnings. The first 3D group had consisted of ten people who were unable to cope with certain aspects of their life. We needed and wanted the support of each other to make course corrections in our lives—diet corrections, money corrections, schedule corrections, spiritual corrections.

Hesitantly at first, and then with increasing confidence, we opened our hearts to one another. And God met us in our honesty and willingness to be vulnerable and to trust Him in the process.

The needs in those first groups were about managing time or losing weight or getting into a disciplined lifestyle with regular prayer times and Bible readings. But there were also big needs—not much different from the grief therapy groups I'd just heard about. I will never forget the sadness and grief we shared with Mary, who had lost her eighteen-year-old son, Jimmy. She couldn't talk about it—she would just sit in our group and cry.

How could one possibly compare the pressure one person was feeling about being overweight with the pressure of grief Mary was feeling? But it worked in a 3D group, the same as it worked in the grieving therapy groups. There is a bond that happens in small groups when people are willing to be open and honest with each other.

My prolonged grief over the loss of Joshua was perfectly acceptable to my family and friends. But I had to work to make it acceptable to myself. One thing for sure: It was making me very soft and needy.

I was not, at that moment, in a 3D group, but I was living the life of 3D. I shared daily with my editor, David; my publisher, Lillian; and several close friends—Lorie, Camie, and Barbara. Like a 3D group, they heard my complaints, monitored my anger and self-pity, and prayed for me.

For weeks David had been saying, "God wants to talk to you, Carol—just listen. Before you write, listen. Sit quietly and listen." Easy for him to say! My deadline loomed so large I wanted to scream every time he said that.

Another journal dialogue went like this:

> I'm really scared about all this writing, Lord. Please give me specific direction of what you want in print.
>
> *I would have you believe in me beyond where you have ever believed in me before.... All that you have been going through has to do with getting "stuff" out of the way of the stream that will flow freely and beautifully from your inner spirit. Your lack of faith and lack of trust in me are the real problems, not your writing ability. If you have life from me, then whatever goes into the book will give life to others. It is not the words, it is not even the story . . . it is my life in you that is needed, not empty words.*

I did regular Bible reading, had quiet time, and even stopped throughout the day for reading and prayer—

wasn't that enough? And keeping a spiritual journal had been a part of my quiet time for years. But David was asking for more. He was encouraging me to just sit in front of my laptop and not write a word until I had first heard from the Lord. This was hard listening. I was goal oriented, an achiever. I took pride in accomplishing a lot of things—all at once. How could I possibly just sit in front of a laptop and pray and not do anything? My quiet time and journal writing were done *before* I got into my day. It was much easier to hear God before the phone started ringing and the family started moving about.

When 3D started in the seventies, there were only a few support groups functioning—with AA being the largest and best known. In Christian circles the small-group movement called Faith at Work pioneered the church scene and started to open doors of communication and caring among church members. Like AA, 3D was dealing with real and practical problems, but it was also like Faith at Work, as prayer and Bible reading were a part of the weekly meetings. 3D was the first faith-based diet program, and it paved the way for the many that were to come on the scene over the next 20 years.

David knew God wanted more of me. And so he pressed me further than I wanted to go. No longer could I separate the God who helped me with my grief and the God who gave me thoughts and ideas for projects. They were one and the same. I could not compartmentalize my life when it came to my relationship with God. There was a time for wisdom, but there was also a time when, like a father, He wanted to enfold me in His arms.

He wanted to walk beside me through the death and grief process with Joshua. He knew every sparrow that fell to the ground, and He knew Joshua was going to die. He knew my pain was real. He knew there was still a residue of grief inside of me because of things in my distant past. And He knew that the experience of grieving for Joshua would touch those areas again and heal them. He was ready to help me.

"My dear Lord," my lips responded, "I have been your child for over forty years. You have been with me in my darkest hours and have blessed me when I have least deserved it. And yet I am still too slow to slip into your arms and rest there at times like these. Forgive me and remind me of what I am missing when I insist on doing things myself. Nudge me in my heart, and cause me to listen to your still small voice."

And then I heard these words in my heart that I wrote on a piece of paper:

> *I am as close as the fingers on your hand, and my spirit lives within you. Our communication can be immediate and direct. There are also times of meditation and contemplation, and times when you should ponder things in your heart before presenting them to me. And there are times when I will not answer immediately. I will always do what is best for you—as any father would do for his children.*

My daily journal was now alive, with sparks flying from every page. No boring entries, no reports of the day's activities. I was asking questions and getting answers. I was feeling His comfort and love deeper than ever. God and I were in a dialogue every single day. Sometimes, when I didn't have time to write in my journal, I would just put my thoughts straight into this book. I would have preferred to keep them private, but it seemed that God intended otherwise. He had brought me face to face with Himself. And in so doing,

He had brought me face to face with myself. He cared about Joshua, me, and the revision of 3D—nothing had to be put aside if I would walk with Him and listen carefully.

These thoughts made me think again about 3D and how all of this related. Isn't the pressure of busy schedules and commitments one of the biggest problems with dieting? Is it possible to separate food problems from emotions? The same old problems plague the dieter: How can I do it all? Diet? Exercise? Work? Family? Sleep? Devotions?

We need the grace of God. We cannot do it in our own strength!

The original book ended in 1975 when I was confronted with leaving God out of the fast-growing 3D program. Guess what: I was doing it again with this revision. Back then He used Cay Andersen and Judy Sorensen to confront me about it. This time He let the circumstances around me drive me to the same place— that of needing to keep Him at the very center of everything I did. Even as I wondered how I would write a chapter to be placed between the old and the new, God had it all worked out.

᠀

Gradually, as my frustration dissipated, gratitude began to fill my heart. My fears were pushed aside, and faith slowly but surely began to reclaim the ground I had lost. Grief and hurt subsided. Love and peace moved in—the indescribable, unfailing love and peace of God.

As if that wasn't enough, God dropped a love gift for me. The doorbell rang, and a florist stood there, holding a beautiful potted plant—actually four different green plants, all different shapes and sizes and shades of green, in one large terra cotta pot. Bursting with signs of new life, within days they would be springing upward and outward. New life was sprouting from every corner.

I opened the card attached to the pink bow. On it was written: "I understand. He must have been greeted by Jonathan. Love, Judy Sorensen."

This was the same Judy who had been so instrumental in my life thirty years before. Her teaching partner, Cay, had died in 1988, and Judy was now retired from active ministry. Her sending her love and care to me over the death of Joshua touched me deeply, as she herself had lost her dog, Jonathan, that had been close to her for many years. And I had no idea she even knew about Joshua. She was a person in my life who had always pointed me to Jesus, well before the beginning of 3D.

Years ago Judy had been talking to me about my judgments, my critical attitude, and my demand for ego satisfaction—all the things I needed to work on in order to grow spiritually. Today she had again met me at a point of great need—ministering this time not with words, but with flowers. Doesn't that sound like a love gift from God?

The 3D book assignment had forced me to depend on the inspiration and direction of the Holy Spirit for thoughts and ideas. The death of my beloved pet forced me to go to Him for comfort and healing.

Only God could have allowed these two things to crash together. I used to be capable of handling multiple crises in my life. In fact, I'd carried that capability as a badge of honor. Carol Showalter didn't cave in easily. But the crying wouldn't stop, and the deadline was getting closer. Unfortunately, when things get to this point in my daily life, I often end up accusing God of putting too much on my plate. I also always run to a friend to ease the pressure and get some answers. Something is wrong with this mode of behavior. And God was requiring me to take action on this account. He was the one who could give me answers. He was the one I needed. Friends were fine—but no one can compare to a Savior.

In my heart I could hear Him saying,

> *You think you can handle everything, as long as it is done in your time and in your way. Then when you can't handle it, somehow it becomes my problem. Turn towards me, and in every single thing I will direct your paths, as I have promised.*

I was learning how to listen to God in a whole new way: Sit, be quiet, and listen. Expect an answer—a *real* answer, not just a weak, gray thought that can barely be discerned. And this is not presumption. It is an attitude of faith and dependency upon a God who has all the answers.

I smiled as I wrote that in my prayer journal. And suddenly I was reminded of that smile face on the room divider in Parkminster Church in Rochester, so long ago. "Smile, God has the answer!" That little slogan had started the 3D program. And now God was telling me the same thing—in a newer and more profound way.

❧

"Dear Lord," I prayed, "help me not to be presumptuous or to demand that you speak every time I throw a question your way. But do give me the faith to believe that it is possible to hear from you specifically and directly about a situation. Free me from accusing you. And help me to trust you when your ways are not my ways."

Another prayer, another answer: Sunday morning, church time. I almost didn't want to go to church because the revision wasn't finished. But what better place to listen to Him than in church? It should actually be easier there than at home or in the office.

My church, the Church of the Transfiguration, is ecumenical. My husband, Bill, is one of the ten ministers on staff. Located as it is at picturesque Rock Harbor on Cape Cod, it draws many visitors in the summer months. This Sunday was no exception. I glanced around as an usher led me to a seat at the end of a row halfway up the church.

Among the visitors a young man wearing a clergy collar stood out. There were five people with him—his three young boys, his wife, and his mother. I recognized the mother—Erin, from Canada. "That's enough looking," I told myself. "Time to get to some serious church business—prayer." I knelt to pray, but not to do my familiar litany of intercession. Instead, I quietly told the Lord that I wanted to hear His voice. I was just going to listen and not talk—a change for me.

Back in the office, my laptop was turned off. But I could not turn off my mind. Like an unruly child, it kept fidgeting and squirming, looking around for thoughts and ideas.

The organ began to play the prelude. By an act of my will, I forced my mind to sit still. "Lord," I thought, "I do feel more peaceful about Joshua. Thank you for that."

My mind was beginning to quiet down. Prayers started to come to my mind and to my lips. "Bless this service, Lord, bless those who pray and sing and preach this morning. Prepare me for communion."

The choir processed in, followed by the clergy. The first hymn was sung. The church was ready to hear God. I felt more ready today than I had in quite some time. "Thank you, Lord."

I did want to hear from God about the book project, and David had suggested an exercise to help me do that when I got stuck during my writing times.

"Just tell the Lord you're sitting there quietly in a movie theater. Ask Him to give you a scene on the screen, and start from there."

I tried that now, attempting to see the next scene for the book. But the screen in my mind stayed blank. I did sense thoughts forming in my heart, however, as the choir sang an anthem. I borrowed a pen from a friend next to me and started writing on that morning's bulletin.

> *This is my house of worship. It is not a theater. Forget your book, and worship me. . . . Listen to me in the Word being read, listen to me in the music being sung, hear me in the preaching, and touch me in Holy Communion. Think on me, my child. I am here. I am walking through this church, touching and loving these people through this service of worship. I am in the rafters. I am in the pews. My dear friend, worship me. Forget yourself.*

Tears came down my cheeks, different from those I'd cried for Joshua. I felt so self-centered. God had given me so much time and patience and love these past twelve days. Why in the world was I doing weekday work on His day, in His house?

For the rest of the service, I focused on Him. And only Him. And He *was* there—in the singing, in the rafters, moving among the congregation, in the prayers, and in Holy Communion.

I remained seated after the postlude had ended and the people had all left. In the ensuing silence I pondered what I'd learned in this most meaningful of Sunday services: that I had so much more to learn!

Finally I left the church, with my spirit lifted, my mind renewed. I had truly had a worship experience. Now I was equipped for a week of service to Him, no matter what I worked on. I used to tell young people, "Just sitting in a church doesn't make you a Christian, any more than sitting in a garage makes you a car." Well, today I had learned that sitting in a worship service doesn't mean you know how to worship. You have to work at it. And it is worth the effort.

❧

I could hardly wait for Monday morning, sensing that this would be a breakthrough week. My plan was to get started early—but something else happened that morning. Van, a ninety-two-year-old friend living with us, had fallen in her room before daylight. She'd been getting ready for an outing to Nantucket with another friend, but instead I would be driving with her to Cape Cod Hospital for stitches in the back of her head. This was not exactly how either of us had planned to start the day.

Van is a remarkable woman. There was no panic in her; she just found all this to be a big inconvenience. I got her comfortable, washed off the blood and cleansed the wound, and then chatted with her to make sure she was really all right. Then I ran across the yard to let a neighbor know we were going to the hospital.

Just as I got to my neighbor's patio, out came Erin from their guesthouse. The day before, I had recognized her in church with the priest.

She didn't ask me what I was doing so early in the morning, and I didn't ask her what she was doing down here from Canada. What she did say, however, blew me away.

"Carol, imagine! Here I am on Cape Cod with my son, who's just been ordained, and his three children and lovely wife. How blessed I am! And all because twenty-five years ago I joined a 3D group to lose weight. That's how it all began, you know!" She laughed. "And now look at me!"

I laughed, too. I looked at her—she was not thin, but she was beaming. This was not the woman I'd met so long ago in the living room of Helen and Bert's house in Toronto, in one of our first 3D leader training seminars in Canada. This was a new woman, alive and vibrant, and thanking God for all her blessings!

Yesterday in church, I had been worried about the next scene for the book, and now I was worried about all the writing time I would lose as I headed for the hospital. Yet here, before my eyes, God was setting the perfect scene—without any effort on my part.

The scene was Toronto, Ontario, in Canada. More than fifty women had gathered in this living room to share the love of God, to encourage each other, and to learn spiritual truths that would set us free to enjoy God and his goodness.

Erin's story was the story of countless thousands of women all over North America over the past thirty years, whose lives have been changed because they joined a Christian diet program.

As I sat in the hospital waiting room while Van was being examined and prepared for getting stitches, my mind went back to that first meeting with Erin.

As Rochester was about four hours from Toronto, Helen and Bert periodically asked me to come up and speak at their leadership meetings. At one particular meeting, I was talking about hurts from the past that bound us and kept us from being free in Christ.

In the back of the room sat a pretty woman I'd not seen before. She asked a few questions during the question-and-answer period, and I noted she had a definite Irish brogue.

"How can God heal hurts that go way back in your childhood?" she wanted to know.

"He's not limited by time or space. He's able to heal anything we bring to Him," I answered.

"That's a little hard to believe," Erin responded honestly.

"It may seem that way, but I can tell you from personal experience, it *is* possible."

After the meeting was over, and everyone was milling around and chatting, Erin made her way to me. Her eyes were brimming.

"Can I talk privately with you?" she asked quietly.

"Of course." I led her to a small den where we could talk.

Twenty-five years later, I can't remember a word of what she shared. But I do remember there were many hurts in her childhood back in Ireland, and she had a bucket full of unforgiveness stored in her heart.

So we started the process of emptying the bucket and inviting God to come in and fill those spaces with His love and His forgiveness. Divorced, with two small children and things not looking promising, Erin was carrying many burdens from her past. She had gained a lot of weight, and her self-worth was at a low ebb.

With the help of her new 3D friends, Erin started to get the help and support she needed. She would remain part of 3D for at least the next ten years.

Our paths crossed numerous times. We often attended the same retreats and special events in Canada and the States. Our children were enrolled in the same Christian school in Canada, and she often came to Cape Cod to visit friends at the Community of Jesus.

Even so, our chance meeting on this particular Monday morning was not chance at all. It was pre-arranged (God arranged), and it reminded me of similar "coincidences." Another lesson in trusting the Lord.

I wouldn't even guess how many needy women like Erin passed through the wide-open doors of Helen and Bert's home. Nor would we ever know just how many lives were dramatically changed by membership in a 3D class in Canada, or for that matter, anywhere in the world.

Van ended up with nine stitches in her head that morning. And I ended up totally renewed by my recalling the miracles of God and by the scene He had given me so easily this morning.

๛

Journalists often call me for interviews and articles on Christian diet programs, of which there are many now. To my delight, 3D is always listed as the first program in this field. A persistent question is this: How does God fit into all of this dieting stuff, or does He?

Recently a reporter asked me if I had any regrets about opening up the whole area of dieting as being a spiritual as well as a physical problem.

I've been thinking a lot about that. Perhaps the problem with the whole weight loss/God concept is that we all want it to be a success story (our idea of a success story). If we love God enough, we will eat properly. If we love God enough, we will be thin. If we memorize our Scripture verses, we will be free from the temptations of our flesh. We want a method that will make us win. A method to stay thin, a method to keep out of depression, a method to manage our time properly.

We are striving for the wrong things. Wholeness in body, mind, and spirit is what we need to strive for. And one without the other makes us off balance. Certainly, there is a lot of attention focused on the body these days. And there is no shortage of thin people in the world—in many cases too thin, as anorexia still wields great power over girls and women between the ages of thirteen and twenty-five. And diet programs and diet products collect literally billions of dollars from men, women, and children seeking to lose weight.

Never have so many people been in counseling, taking medications for depression and anxieties, or been involved with therapy groups. The mind is in trouble and people are seeking help everywhere they can get it.

It's the spirit that is lagging behind the trends of today, allowing the cart to pull the horse.

3D began a trend—one of matching up body, mind, and spirit. It's still a proven combination for wholeness.

I believe that bringing God into this whole equation makes it a win-win situation. Nothing is ever wasted with Him, and He can use all things in our lives. He has asked us to care for one another and most especially to pray for one another. We need to be faithful to the Scriptures, and we need to give glory to God in our bodies. With these goals in mind beyond a weight goal, you will be a winner!

⁀

The incident with Erin gave me thoughts of many people across the United States and Canada who had become friends over the telephone and through newsletters. Why not pick up the phone and call some of them? But before making even one call, I prayed. Then I sat still and listened. And I wrote down the names that came to me in that quiet time.

The first person I talked to was Roberta in California. About five months before, she had written me a letter that had touched my heart, about her daughter, Nicole. When Roberta first joined 3D in the 1980s, we received a call to pray for Nicole, who was born with heart problems. We were faithful in our prayers. Nicole is now sixteen, and Roberta wanted to thank the 3D office for their many prayers. Just this year, Nicole was given her first clean bill of health and does not need to check in for one year.

Then I called Mary Lou, a parish nurse in Ohio. A paper was presented to a convention of parish nurses ten years ago, and the presenter was Mary Lou. This paper presented 3D as the best program for overall wholeness for churches to be involved in. She wrote pages and pages of data about the value of a program such as this. (Her paper is available on 3D's Web site for you to read.) Mary Lou is still a big fan of 3D and continues to recommend it for everyone. From the time of that presentation until now, 3D continues to be a valuable tool in the hands of parish nurses all over the country. And 3D exhibits at their national convention. "It is one our favorite conventions," says Laura in our sales department, "and they all love 3D." Thanks, Mary Lou!

In making calls to individuals around the country I also wanted to talk to some of the original 3D members from Parkminster church. For Mary Jane, now the grandmother of four, weight continues to be a big struggle. But she has never given up. Last year she was diagnosed with diabetes and was put on insulin. But perseverance is her middle name. Three months ago she started again, this time riding her bicycle every day. I just spoke to her. She has lost 30 pounds, and her doctor has taken her off insulin.

Jan, living now in Chandler, Arizona, was the next contact I made. She'd been a 3D leader for many years. "Carol, to tell you the truth, I have wonderful memories from our 3D groups, and I still keep in touch with women from those first groups. The friendships started there have been lifelong, and even when I haven't talked with someone for several years, it feels like we can just pick up and talk again, as if the miles and years between us don't exist." I felt this way, talking to her. We'd not visited for years, and yet it was like we were sitting over a cup of tea at the manse in Rochester.

She paused, and then added, "I think the biggest problem I carried around from those groups was the disappointment in myself, that I never lost much weight. I felt guilty about that. After all, as a leader of a Christian diet program, shouldn't I have been more successful in the weight department?"

"I understand exactly what you're saying, Jan," I smiled. "I'd dare say there are hundreds of people who have felt the same way over the years—including me." I thought for a moment. "Perhaps in the early days, thinness *was* our goal. But as the years went on, we realized that weight was only a small part of the program. As I read testimonies today, I hear much more about the drive to lose the weight in our first timers. But Jan, it's all right. God knows exactly how to get our attention, and He works with what means the most to us. The first D in 3D is Diet, so we start there."

Sensing that whatever Jan might share would certainly be helpful to others, I asked her if she would write a testimony for the book.

"I'd love to write something for you, because God certainly used that time in my life in a deep and tremendous way." Then she laughed. "And remember, I found my husband right there in that church at that time. We just celebrated our twenty-ninth anniversary!"

Who knew what plan God had for Jan back then? Was getting thin the number one priority? I doubt it. Did she, as a registered nurse, help a lot of people in those groups? You bet she did! Was her life in Christ a blessing to others? Absolutely. And she found her husband, too. Successful? I'd say so.

The calls went on, and the stories were incredible. More than once I found myself in tears. I talked to Bev, Jo, Mary, Tom, Jane, Dorcas, and many others—people from the early groups. Some of the testimonies will be found in this book, others on the Web site. All will just serve as reminders and blessings to me and to the 3D staff about the power of the 3D program to change lives. As for helping people achieve thinness, 3D may have about the same "success rate" as other diet groups. But one thing is certain: It can boast in the power of Jesus Christ to transform lives. That was what it was about in the seventies—and that is what it is about in the new millennium.

❧

I looked out the garage office window as I was finishing this update. The scene had changed. The sun was just hitting the tall stalks of corn in our garden, with husks and strains of silk flowing out of them. And to the left were the beautiful yellow, orange, white, and passion-red gladioli. Several of them were so laden with blossoms that they were leaning over into the garden, bumping their beautiful blossoms up against the tomato stakes. Tomatoes were poking their heads out of the vines with bright red faces. Colors everywhere—a bright yellow finch flew in and out of the trees and perched atop the fence.

A little further to the left was the miniature pine tree. It looked so sweet under those big pines. It, too, was being hit by the new morning rays of sun. That same spot that had given me so much pain a few weeks before was now blessing me. God had done a work in my soul. I would never be the same because of the new spiritual journey the Lord had taken me through.

At that moment I realized this was all the plan of God. He knew what should be in the book. He knew what I needed in my life. And He would, if I let Him, bring it all together. I had to write about this because it spoke of an honest struggle that I was having in the summer of 2001. When I wrote the original *3D* book in 1977, I was struggling with my weight, struggling with my fear of being a minister's wife, struggling with my jealousies and my need for acceptance. And I was struggling to forgive myself for just being a plain old sinner. I still struggle—and God remains ever faithful. *This is my story.*

❧

In these pages you have walked with me through different levels of hurt and pain. You have let me share with you my questioning, my wrestling with God, and His answers to me. You have been a part of a new beginning in my life—as God directed me and spoke to me as I wrote. You have been in my quiet time and you have been with me as I journaled.

As we look forward to a new burst of excitement and energy that is going to come forth through the 3D program, remember that God has not called us to "get better" or to "get thinner." He has called us to know Him and to know ourselves. This will take each of us a lifetime.

But believe me, it's a lot more fun doing it with a support group around you!

TESTIMONIES

In the next few pages I want you to meet some of the 3D family, both from the first days and from new groups. The testimonies of what God has done in their lives will bless your own life. And if you wouldn't mind, do me a favor: Send me your own testimony after you have completed the first twelve weeks of the program, so we can rejoice with you in the faithfulness of God.

Dear God, protect this program called 3D.
Keep it always centered on you and your Word.
May it always bring glory to your name. Amen.

Renee Vigoroso

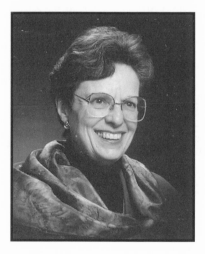

*I*n 1977 I joined my first 3D group at my church in Cambridge, Massachusetts, and I have continued to be involved as member, leader and area coordinator. This fall there are eight eager women ready to do session one. 3D has become part of my spiritual life, and I am grateful.

What I have always found is that people need to learn a new way of life from and through Jesus Christ, and to learn the importance and place of discipline and discipleship in the process.

As far as weight is concerned, all my life I thought I was overweight. When I was young, I went to an obesity doctor, had the shot, took the diuretics, and lost 20 pounds. And when I joined 3D, my goal was to lose those 20 pounds again.

Guess what? I still felt internally anesthetized against feelings; I was quiet and kept to myself, and one of the saddest things was that I really wasn't aware there was another way to live. The weight loss didn't change a thing. There was other work to be done in my life. With the help of God, my husband, and my 3D friends, things changed for me. I am a different person.

Building habits of obedience in my thought life, in the words I speak, and in my actions seems to have built in me a greater sense of security in Jesus rather than in my self-sufficiency.

Special 3D friends for life now live in Germany, Maine, Rhode Island, and Massachusetts. We stay in touch. This richness in relationship that comes from being freed from hindrances that used to keep me isolated from people is probably the great gift Jesus, through 3D, has given me.

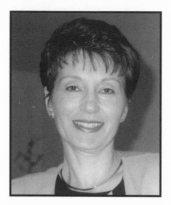

Karen Wyatt

I really didn't know anything about the 3D program when I joined. However, I had been in another church-related diet group several years before. I had found that when I try to lose weight on my own without a support system, it just doesn't work.

Our leader is a nurse, so she had training in many aspects of health. But you see, this program is not just for someone wanting to take off some pounds. It is for someone who wants to grow in his or her walk with the Lord, have fellowship with others, and learn the disciplines of a spiritual life.

My group supports and encourages each other, and there is a sense of family as each one is working and committing to a similar goal. One of the special blessings is a time of prayer, where each of those present prays for other members of the group. There are many unexpected benefits and blessings in this program. I hope you will discover them too.

Patti Wagner

The healing and reconciliation ministry team of our United Methodist church in Virginia found on a church-wide survey that many of our members were struggling with weight control problems. After researching many of the popular weight loss programs, our parish nurse chose to offer the 3D program. The attraction of the program was its holistic approach not just to weight loss, but to an overall healthy lifestyle. We wanted to have not just the physical aspects of the program, but also the aspects of emotional, relational, and spiritual well-being included in what we did.

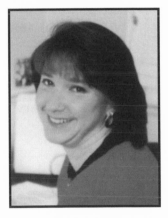

Our church is committed to assisting its members to be whole persons in Christ. We are thankful for what this program has done for our members. We will continue to offer new classes in hopes that more people will come to know what it means to be a healthy Christian.

Here are two short testimonies from members of this church:

Nita Lewis

I wish to say how much the 3D classes meant to me. First, I began to see many things that I had not paid close attention to as a Christian. So many subjects really opened my eyes. 3D made me wish to be a better person and to show love and concern for my fellow man. Next, I was a great deal overweight, and the diet did a lot to push me in the right direction. I lost 30 pounds, and it made me feel better mentally as well as physically.

Carol Trott

*B*eing a part of the 3D program was a great experience. The devotions helped me to realize that I do need God to achieve my goals, and I have to be willing to ask for help. Even though I completed the twelve weeks with a successful loss of fifteen pounds, I consider this to be an ongoing program for me.

Len and Pat Harding

Len:

*H*ere I was in my seventies and the 3D meditation was on *growing*. Now that was humorous! But as I started to write this testimony, I realized that growth was what I needed. I found that I was dwelling on things in the past, recalling past failures, not forgiving myself. Jesus was faithful and He was forgiving, but I

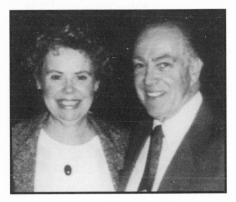

could never forgive myself. In my daily thoughts I would get the prodding to pray more, to get into God's Word, to be more conscious of God in my life. I needed healing for the past.

It is interesting to look back on my beginnings in 3D. God knew my every thought, and yet I was afraid to let my thoughts become known to Him. I guess that was because if I *really* let God know my thoughts, that process would reveal to me who I really am.

3D reminded me that God loves us. He called us to share our life in Christ with others. As I continued in 3D, I became aware of how God brought me into contact with some very wonderful friends, friends with whom I could share my fears, my feelings, my hopes.

Participating in the 3D chat line on the Internet is a real blessing. I expressed a desire to write in my retirement. With promises of prayer I was encouraged to give it a try. Since that time I have had three articles published in newspapers and magazines, and three more accepted for publication. 3D has been a definite plus in my life.

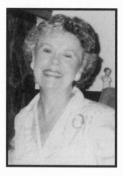

Pat:

*I*n my forties my body was changing along with my figure. As a Christian I was attracted to a Christian diet program called 3D. Through my fifties and sixties I continued in 3D groups, always receiving encouraging truth about fats, calories, exercises, and much, much more. The devotionals, weekly memory verses, and prayer fed and supported me, teaching me that old habits can be changed.

Learning about myself—where and why was I angry, depressed, insecure, and fearful—I truly found new life with fresh and wholesome goals and aims. I had many breakthroughs and healings in the program.

Now I am in my seventies, and I continue to need reality and growth and change. Thanks to modern technology, I now receive help through the online 3D chat room.

Roberta Riggs

*J*oined 3D in Vallejo, California, and attended my first real Bible study ever. I had two young sons, and I found that 3D was just what I needed. It was not only the diet, but also the fellowship and learning about God and myself that were so special to me, and I just loved it all. Then I became pregnant with Nicole and was bedridden during that time. Nicole was born in 1984, and we found out 30 minutes after her birth that some-

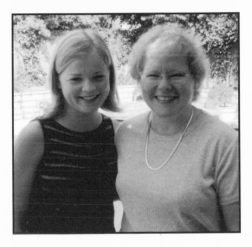

thing was terribly wrong with her heart. She was missing the right lower chamber of her heart and would require open-heart surgery in the first two days after she was born. It was not likely that her life span was going to be long. We were told that five years would be a lot for her.

The road ahead was very rough. We went through the surgery followed by large doses of medication, and many hospital stays just to control the infection that was always ready to attack.

About the time Nicole was nine months old, people began to ask me about starting a new 3D group. When I called to order the materials, Carol asked how I was, and I began to tell her about Nicole and her condition. She said she would put our situation on the bulletin board at work so that Nicole would be prayed for daily by the 3D staff. No matter when I called in the weeks and months that followed, I was always asked how Nicole was doing. With all the stress on me I could barely pray. To know that people all over the United States were praying for our little girl meant everything to me and to my family.

We moved away to Sacramento, and quite a while later I started another 3D group there. When I called to order materials, the first question asked of me after all that time was, "How is Nicole doing?" I could not believe it! I knew that the Lord was showing me the love the 3D people had for our family.

God has taken care of us all in mighty ways, and we have learned so much. But I will always remember that the 3D staff was holding us up in prayer, and that they never forgot the family that had been told their daughter would not live past five years of age. Nicole is now sixteen and is doing well.

Barbara Cole

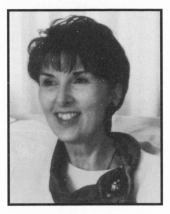

3D was the beginning of my spiritual life and walk. I often think of the banner that once hung at a 3D conference. It used Philippians 3:14: "I press on toward the goal for the prize of the upward call of God in Christ Jesus." This seemed like an appropriate theme for 3D. As I look back on those early days, I can see that through 3D God was planning and leading me to a closer and deeper walk with Him. How would I ever know in those days what His plan was for me? But I took one step at a time, and I continue doing that now, always striving to keep my eyes on Jesus, not on myself or on others.

As I pray, sitting here on the beach writing this testimony, I think, "Why, God, in your mercy and goodness did you allow me to be privileged to know You and to be called to be enveloped in 3D?" And I seem to hear Him reply, "Why, my child, because left to your own devices you would not do My will, but you would become a worldly creature—because that is your human bent. I have saved you from that and have better things for you. Why? Not because I love you more than others, but because you were bent toward Me and allowed that soft side to come to Me."

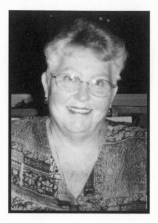

Janice Brule

*M*any years have gone by since I attended my first 3D meeting at Parkminster Presbyterian Church, but the truths I learned there are still working in my life.

Caring for others was the essence of 3D: praying for one another, listening to each other, and actively doing for others as the women expressed their needs.

I am still doing these things as a retired person in my community.

I began to truly trust God to do the work within me, even when I felt no different. Slowly and sometimes over a period of years, I began to feel differently about certain people needing forgiveness. I realized then God really does change me from the inside; all He needed was my willingness to let Him do it.

Dorcas Thompson

The 3D program has left an indelible mark in my life and in my walk with Christ. Aside from the many pleasant memories of friendships, several things stand out in my mind. One of the key elements was the need to fight some things which hampered me from fulfilling God's call on my life. I came to realize that life is a daily conflict between the spirit and the flesh, and that I would have to commit myself to a day by day determination to obey Jesus Christ. I learned, too, the necessity of accountability. It is easy for us to be "Lone Rangers" and try to reach maturity by ourselves. It became vital for me to share myself with sisters in Christ and open myself to them as a way of growing in faith.

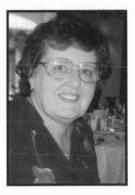

My involvement in 3D was a powerful force in developing my leadership in the care of women. As a pastor's wife, I had been ill-prepared to work alongside my husband. Through work as a 3D co-leader, I learned to enjoy ministering to women and yoke-teaching.

Finally, I learned perseverance! You just "keep on keeping on" and never give up. How necessary that lesson would become in local congregations through the years.

Through the past 25 years I have often found myself grateful for the things added to my life through 3D.

Mary Jane Preston

What has my life been like since I met the Lord in that first 3D group? The truth is that God changed my life, and it has never been the same since.

As 3D grew at our church, I became involved writing materials, planning conferences, and meeting with 3D groups at other churches. It was a busy time and sometimes a bit overwhelming, but the one thing I really learned was that God was in charge of my life. I had always been a person who had goals and who planned ahead to meet them. You can get yourself into a lot of control that way, and sometimes that can feel good. But gradually I began to see the joy of God's surprises. He had better experiences in store for me than I ever could have planned for myself—it was an adventure day by day!

I would like to say that I gained total victory over my weight, and that I have stayed a reasonable weight for the past thirty years. I cannot say that. It has been a constant, and sometimes losing, battle. I did learn basic good nutrition, and that has stood me in good stead over the years. At times it has made me mad that my "problem" is such an obvious one, but God has known what would drive me to him.

Many wonderful things have grown out of my time in 3D. I began to learn how to be a better mother to my son, to my adopted daughter, and to the many foster children who have lived with us over the years. 3D helped my husband and me develop our relationship, and our lives became centered in our church community— what a difference that has made! Our life-long friendships have been with the men and women that we met at church in 3D groups. Instead of just being a good church-going lady, I have learned about a true relationship with Jesus. That first group was a defining moment in my life, and I am so grateful.

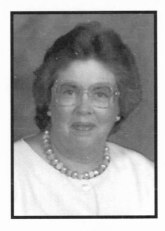

Renee Economides

When 3D came into my life about 15 years ago, I was very frustrated over a weight gain. Even though I had a college degree with an emphasis in nutrition, I became caught up in "fad" diets. After two sessions in 3D, I lost the weight and gained discipline in other areas of my life. I began spending more time in Bible study and prayer, and really grew closer to the Lord as well as feeling better physically. My enthusiasm over the 3D program encouraged me to become an area coordinator to help organize new groups in my city. I had always loved to exercise and decided to start a low-impact aerobics group at my church about 12 years ago, which I continue to teach. Starting new 3D

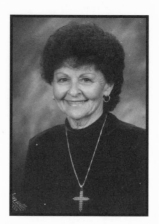

groups, training leaders, and continuing to lead groups has blessed my life with many new friends. I've learned that the prayer support and encouragement of my 3D groups is vital to my spiritual growth, and the 3D disciplines have become a way of life for me.

Roz Pirozzoli Donnelly

I have been on every diet known to man. None has escaped me. . . . I called out to God on a regular basis, "Oh, Lord, after this third slice of pizza, I need to diet. Help me." It was just words, I never meant it; but now I know that God himself heard me.

A friend told me all about 3D, and the following Tuesday my husband drove with me 60 miles each way for the meeting. I took Session 2 back to my area; the group is doing well, and we plan to continue a weekly meeting at my house. We are getting stronger and more disciplined, and learning to care and share. The companionship is great; we never need feel we are alone again.

Rina

*T*his is a first time experience for me of a diet program of this nature. Learning how to eat right, exercise, and stay fit are only part of it. Daily devotions are an important aspect of putting God as first priority, then all else will follow, and it does. The best way to describe 3D is a loving, Christ-centered endeavor that encompasses more than just weight management—it is a way to live.

Dorothy Vitale

*T*he 3D progam has brought the balance my life has needed in order to function in good health—emotionally, physically, and spiritually. Meeting together, our group creates the atmosphere of caring and sharing, the love of Jesus, and promotes the willingness to grow in the Lord. I am forever grateful to my Lord Jesus Christ for giving us this beautiful program.

Antoinette Kelly

*T*he 3D program has helped me tremendously, not only in losing weight, but in discipline and obedience in other areas of my life. Sometimes the program seems so simple and easy to follow I just can't believe it, but I know that God is the reason. The times that I do have a problem is when I am not obedient and try to do things my way. Not only have I lost weight, but I am grateful that I have lost some bad habits and bad attitudes.

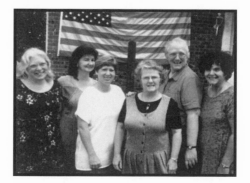

3D
The Program

Welcome to the 3D Program

3D is a faith-based support group. Although it is possible to go through the program as an individual, it is our recommendation that you ask at least one other person to share this journey with you. Encouragement and accountability to someone else are keys to a successful venture.

The following pages will discuss the basic components of the program and will give you, in detail, the information necessary for you to receive help in three areas—diet, discipline, and discipleship. This is a guidebook, a member's manual, to assist you along the way. Read through every page and begin the process of charting your course. Twelve weeks is the recommended time commitment you need to make. The program has been put together in twelve-week segments.

You will need to order your devotional book from 3D (1-800-451-5006), or purchase it from your local bookstore. *Devotions for Daily Living* will give you a daily Bible reading, a devotional on the particular theme of the week, and questions. This is the core of the program—a very essential ingredient.

May God bless your life as you seek to be wholly His—body, soul, and spirit.

3D Benefits

Physical
☑ A well-balanced diet program from the American Dietetic and Diabetic Association.
☑ The use of daily exercise to promote the well-being of God's temple—your body.

Spiritual
☑ Bible readings and questions.
☑ Daily devotional readings.
☑ Scripture memorization.
☑ Growth, both individually and as a group.

Emotional
☑ Understanding yourself better.
☑ Sharing through small groups that meet weekly.
☑ Caring for others.

Social
☑ Reaching out within churches, neighborhoods, and communities.
☑ Getting to know people of different ages and backgrounds.
☑ Learning to be at ease with yourself and with others.

We believe this program will provide the ABCs you need to become a better you!

Begin with anticipation! God bless you as you begin this new adventure!

Healthy Eating

The diet part of this program introduces you to a plan for sensible eating habits. 3D has successfully helped over half a million people learn the value of good eating. Healthy eating has become an increasing need in our society where fast foods have become a daily habit instead of a treat once in a while. We find ourselves "driving through" to get our breakfast, lunch, or dinner on our way to something else. Family mealtime happens only once or twice a week instead of daily.

God has always used the area of food to teach his people truth about themselves and about him. The Garden of Eden is our first introduction to the individual wanting to do "his/her" own thing when it came to eating! "I want what I want when I want it" is the cry that came out of the garden and is still the cry of most of us when it comes to food.

The manna from heaven was provided by God to show his people that he did care about their hunger, and that he would indeed take care of them. But soon the manna didn't satisfy (does that sound familiar?). Then, of course, throughout the life of Jesus many of

His miracles centered around food—the feeding of the 5,000, the wedding feast at Cana and others. His teaching often occurred around the table—with Martha and Mary, with Zacchaeus, and of course with His disciples. Jesus' very life is given to us by our receiving the bread and wine in Communion. And, at the end of life, we have all been invited to the banquet table with Him. Food is woven in and out of the Bible with great significance, and it is woven in and out of our lives today in much the same way.

Food, like everything else, needs to come under the Lordship of Christ, and we need to walk towards that goal. The whole area of food brings out rebellion, fear, and anxiousness, and it reveals a lot about who we are inside (which is exactly what happened in the Bible!).

In 3D we are concerned with sound nutrition and well-balanced meals, and we would like to thank Pamela Saltsman, M.P.H., R.D., for her contribution to this revised edition of the Member's Manual. We have used the ADA (American Dietetic Association) diet as the basis of our program. The calories have already been counted and the individual is taught about the basic food groups and about how to exchange foods within groups. Once you learn the ADA diet, it is always a part of your thinking.

If you have joined a group for the purpose of losing weight, we believe the ADA diet is a medically sound diet plan. If you have joined to get help with anorexia nervosa and need to gain weight, we also believe the ADA plan is the best instruction you can receive to help you with your eating disorder. If you have joined any group sponsored by 3D and are not at all interested in dieting, please consider acquainting yourself with this plan. We believe it will be a tremendous blessing to you and your family and will be a real aid to better health.

Looking at food with the following exchange lists in mind is a new experience, and it takes practice to become familiar with them. So don't be discouraged, and do allow time for menu planning.

The 3D program emphasizes good nutrition, proper eating habits and sensible weight loss. While you are in this program, the whole family can benefit from well-balanced meals and will develop good eating habits. They can eat all the same foods you do, adding extras like larger servings or sauces.

3D's Dietitian

Loretta Jack, R.D., is a Registered Dietitian with the American Dietetic Association. Ms. Jack has a Bachelor of Science degree from Cornell University in food and nutrition. She completed her dietetic internship at Massachusetts General Hospital. For nine years she continued to work there, first as a staff therapeutic dietitian, and then as unit coordinator for the medical building.

Charting Your Course

As you consider what your weight is and what you want it to be, do remember that the following charts and equations are only guidelines, and that you should prayerfully consider what is right for you.

Many people have strong feelings about what their ideal weight is, but their opinion may differ from what is right for them. For example, a person who has lost weight may wish to continue to the point where he or she becomes excessively thin. Then it is important for someone to help the person examine whatever feelings may be underneath this desire.

By using the Harris-Benedict equation on page 184, you can adjust your daily caloric intake to meet your weight loss or weight maintenance needs. Once you have determined how many calories you need to eat each day, find the exchanges for this number of calories in the chart on the Model Meal Plan (see page 189). Watch your weight carefully, although not obsessively, as you begin the new diet. Each person's body reacts differently, and further adjustments may be needed.

One advantage of the 3D diet is that it trains members in proper eating habits. Eating habits developed during weight loss (or weight gain) are the basis for the disciplined eating that should continue throughout life.

As members begin a maintenance regimen, they will continue to learn how they can manage their food intake so they won't gain back the weight they lost. Members will learn how many extras they can have or how much larger their portions can be. Even on maintenance regimen the same good habits of low-fat, high-fiber eating will be reinforced.

Lactating and pregnant women should check with their doctor before beginning any diet program.

WHAT'S THE RIGHT WEIGHT?

Ideal body weight differs for each person. Each person has her or his own unique body composition based on body frame and distribution of fat and muscle. The location and amount of fat are sometimes better predictors than actual body weight for determining a person's health risk. For example, a muscular person may seem to be overweight according to weight charts. But, because muscle weighs more than fat, the person may actually be at his proper weight.

The Body Mass Index or BMI is a standard measurement that researchers use to assess obesity. You can calculate your BMI by dividing your weight (in kilograms) by your height (in meters) squared. Or use the chart below to estimate your BMI.

		Body Mass Index (BMI)												
		19	20	21	22	23	24	25	26	27	28	29	30	35	40
		Weight (pounds)													
	4'10"	91	96	100	105	110	115	119	124	129	134	138	143	167	191
	4'11"	94	99	104	109	114	119	124	128	133	138	143	148	173	198
	5'0"	97	102	107	112	118	123	128	133	138	143	148	153	179	204
	5'1"	100	106	111	116	122	127	132	137	143	148	153	158	185	211
	5'2"	104	109	115	120	126	131	136	142	147	153	158	164	191	218
	5'3"	107	113	118	124	130	135	141	146	152	158	163	169	197	225
	5'4"	110	116	122	128	134	140	145	151	157	163	169	174	204	232
Height	5'5"	114	120	126	132	138	144	150	156	162	168	174	180	210	240
	5'6"	118	124	130	136	142	148	155	161	167	173	179	186	216	247
	5'7"	121	127	134	140	146	153	159	166	172	178	185	191	223	255
	5'8"	125	131	138	144	151	158	164	171	177	184	190	197	230	262
	5'9"	128	135	142	149	155	162	169	176	182	189	196	203	236	270
	5'10"	132	139	146	153	160	167	174	181	188	195	202	207	243	278
	5'11"	136	143	150	157	165	172	179	186	193	200	208	215	250	286
	6'0"	140	147	154	162	169	177	184	191	199	206	213	221	258	294
	6'1"	144	151	159	166	174	182	189	197	204	212	219	227	265	302
	6'2"	148	155	163	171	179	186	194	202	210	218	225	233	272	311
	6'3"	152	160	168	176	184	192	200	208	216	224	232	240	279	319
	6'4"	156	164	172	180	189	197	205	213	221	230	238	246	287	328
								OVERWEIGHT					OBESE		

Source: World Health Organization

The American Institute for Cancer Research (AICR) recommends that people maintain a BMI between 18.5 and 25 throughout their life. The AICR also suggests that people do not gain more than eleven pounds throughout their adult life. Those people with a BMI above 25 are usually defined as "overweight" and those above 30 as "obese."

The BMI overall is a good guideline for determining whether a person is within his or her ideal body weight. However, the BMI is not a good indicator for fat distribution. Therefore, even if your BMI is in a healthy range you may benefit from losing a little weight because your body fat may still be too high. People who have a higher distribution of fat around the chest or belly areas versus their hips and thighs have a higher risk for disease. One way to know if you are carrying excess body fat is through the Waist to Hip ratio.

To determine your Waste to Hip ratio simply divide your waist measurement by your hip measurement. For women, your waist to hip measurement should be at or below 0.85 and for men, 0.95.

How to Set Your Course

You may compute your Daily Caloric Need following the guidelines on these pages. How many calories people require is based on many factors including their age, height, present weight, and activity level.

Your Basal Energy Expenditure (BEE) reflects the number of calories needed when the body is at rest. Once you determine your BEE, you can factor in your activity level to estimate how many calories you burn each day.

Use the Harris-Benedict Equation (1919) below to find out how many calories you need to maintain your weight.

Fill in the blank boxes and compute.

Conversions: weight in pounds ÷ 2.2 = weight in kilograms (kg) height in inches x 2.54 = height in centimeters (cm)

FEMALES:

BEE =   655 + 9.6 x wt(Kg) + 1.8 x ht(cm) – 4.7 x
          age(years)

BEE =   655 + (9.6 x □□ .□) + (1.8 x □□□) – 4.7 x
          □□ = □□□□ Kcal/day

MALES:

BEE =   66 + 13.7 x wt(Kg) + 5 x ht(cm) – 6.7 x
          age(years)

BEE =   66 + (13.7 x □□ .□) + (5 x □□□) – 6.7 x
          □□ = □□□□ Kcal/day

ADJUSTMENT IN BODY WEIGHT FOR OVERWEIGHT PEOPLE:

If you weigh more than 125% of your ideal body weight use the following formula to determine your weight in pounds for the Harris-Benedict equation.

{[Actual body weight – Ideal body weight (IBW)] x 0.25} + IBW =

LIFE STYLE ACTIVITY FACTORS*		
Activity Category		**Activity Factor**
Very Light (sedentary)	seated work minimal or no exercise	1.3–1.4
Light	mostly seated work irregular exercise	1.5
Moderate	seated and lightly active work some regular activity but little strenuous exercise	1.6–1.7
Extremely Active	strenuous work heavy exercise	1.8–2.2

* Adapted from Shetty P.S., et al., 1996 and FAO/WHO/UNO, 1985 and Food & Nutrition Board, National Research Council, NAS, 1989 and National Academy Press, 1989.

Identify your Life Style Activity Factor (see chart above) and multiply by your BEE to find your daily energy need. Most people fall between the light and moderate activity factors. Pray to find the right activity factor for you.

1 497

1.0

Total Energy Requirement = ☐☐☐☐ Kcals/day x ☐.☐
Activity Factor

2359.2

Your Total Energy Requirement tells you how many calories you need for maintenance. To gain or lose weight, you must add or subtract calories from this maintenance level. To lose weight subtract the amounts below, and to gain, add the same amounts.

+/- 500 calories for 1lb/wk weight loss.

+/- 750 calories for 1½lb/wk weight loss.

+/- 1000 calories for 2 lb/wk weight loss.

For weight loss: *Do not drop below 1000 calories/day.*

BEFORE YOU BEGIN

Now that you have established your weight loss (or weight gain) goals, it is important to keep in mind that weight loss, gain, or maintenance cannot be achieved by diet alone. There are three components to forming and keeping healthy habits.

These are:

1. good nutrition
2. exercise
3. behavior modification

Through diet, discipline, and discipleship, 3D helps members work all three components into their life style.

Try to approach the 3D program as a better, healthier way to live your life, rather than "just another diet program." By doing so, you can minimize feelings of deprivation or urges to "cheat." By focusing on healthier habits, rather than on the bathroom scale, you are more likely to be successful in reaching your goals.

LET'S TALK NUTRITION

The USDA, as well as the American Institute for Cancer Research, promotes a low-fat, high-fiber diet. We know that by improving our weight status, avoiding fats, and eating a diet rich in vegetables, fruits, and whole grains, we can help reduce the risk of heart disease, diabetes, and cancer. As always, the 3D program is at the cutting edge of what we know about diet and disease. By using the exchange lists that follow, in combination with using food labels to monitor fat and fiber intake, we can easily achieve a low-fat, high-fiber meal plan.

The Exchange Lists

The Exchange Lists divide our basic food requirements into six categories: Milk, Vegetables, Fruit, Starch, Meat, and Fat. Foods are placed in the categories according to similar vitamin, mineral, carbohydrate, protein, and fat content. Each group provides its own particular type of nutrients, and we need a balance of all the groups for good nutrition. Within each category, the portion size for each exchange is important.

The Exchange Lists reflect the latest thinking in the area of nutrition, based on concern for total caloric intake and for modification of fat.

List 1: *Starch Exchanges* include breads, cereals, grains, pasta, beans, peas and lentils, and starchy vegetables.

List 2: *Fruit Exchanges* give the serving sizes for fruit and fruit juices.

List 3: *Milk Exchanges* include most dairy products.

List 4: *Vegetable exchanges* include all vegetables except starchy vegetables.

List 5: *Meat Exchanges* include not only meat, but also other protein-rich foods.

List 6: *Fat Exchanges* have been revised to show the differences in the kinds of fat.

THE EXCHANGES

We have been talking about "Exchange Lists," and you may ask—"What exactly are they?" When we say "exchange," we mean "substitute." Within each food group, if you do not want one food, you may substitute another. But only substitute foods within a given group—i.e., green beans instead of tomatoes. (You cannot substitute green beans for orange juice.)

It is important to weigh and measure your food according to the amounts listed, as we are very much deceived by our own eyes. (It is amazing to measure a 2-inch apple and see how small it is!) This self-deception is especially noticeable in the Fat Exchange List. By habit, we use much more butter or margarine than we realize and need—one teaspoon of margarine for toast is not very much! Fats are also a source of many calories; for instance, a teaspoon of butter or margarine has twice as many calories as a teaspoon of sugar.

If you are already familiar with the Exchange Lists, the Meat Group will represent a change. As stated above, meats can contain many calories of fat, and they are one of the reasons for greater clarification in the meat group—for extra lean-, lean- and medium-fat meats. A high-fat meat list is not included because these meats should almost never be eaten. It would be easy to actually gain weight by eating too much high-fat meat. So remember, if you eat medium- or high-fat meat, you need to count the extra grams of fat so that you can keep within your daily fat allowance.

You may have noticed that when we get older our caloric needs decrease. Additional exercise does help, but you may well need help readjusting your eating habits from your teens and twenties.

As previously mentioned, we receive calories (energy) from the proteins, fats, and carbohydrates in foods—starches and sugar being the most common carbohydrates. Protein yields amino acids and nitrogen, which are necessary for life, and fat provides a very concentrated source of calories. Vitamins and various minerals are present in all of the food groups, which is why we need a *balance of all the food groups* in our daily diet to have good health.

The 3D diet is not new, but our approach to dieting takes on a new slant when we ask Jesus to help us "exchange" some of our old eating habits for new ones.

MODEL MEAL PLAN
Use the following chart as a guideline for incorporating the exchanges into your daily routine. The exchanges are divided into small meals with snacks. Eating regularly will help prevent cycles of hunger and overeating as well as give your body the energy it needs throughout the day. If necessary, you may adapt this plan to your own life style. However, as you rearrange exchanges and meals, remember to keep meals balanced, and to not space meals too far apart.

Exchanges	Calories per day							
	1000	1200	1500	1800	2000	2400	2600	3000
Breakfast								
Meat			1	1	1	1	1	2
Bread	1	1	1	2	2	3	3	4
Fruit	1	1	1	1	1	1	2	2
Milk	1	1	1	1	1	1	1	1
Fat						1	2	2
Lunch								
Meat	2	3	3	3	3	4	4	4
Bread	1	2	2	2	3	3	3	3
Vegetable	2	2	2	2	2	2	2	2
Fruit				1	1	2	2	2
Milk								
Fat	1	1	1	1	1	2	2	2
Snack								
Meat								
Bread				1	1	2	2	3
Vegetable		1	1	1	1	1	2	2
Fruit	1	1	1	1	1	1	1	2
Milk	1	1	1	1	1	1	1	1
Dinner								
Meat	3	3	3	4	4	4	4	5
Bread	2	2	2	2	3	3	4	4
Vegetable	2	2	2	2	2	2	2	3
Fruit								1
Milk								
Fat		2	2	2	2	2	2	2
Snack								
Bread			1	1	1	1	1	1
Fruit			1	1	1	1	1	1
Milk					1	1	1	1

List 1: Starch Exchanges

Cereals, grains, pasta, breads, crackers, snacks, starchy vegetables, and cooked beans, peas, and lentils are starches. In general, one starch is:

- ½ cup of cereal, grain, pasta, or starchy vegetable,
- 1 ounce of a bread product, such as 1 slice of bread,
- ¾ to 1 ounce of most snack foods. (Some snack foods may also have added fat.)

One starch exchange equals:
- 15 grams carbohydrate,
- 3 grams protein,
- 0-1 grams fat, and
- 80 calories.

BREAD

Bagel	1½ (1 oz)
Bread, reduced-calorie	2 slices (1½ oz)
Bread, white, whole-wheat, pumpernickel, rye	1 slice (1 oz)
Bread sticks, crisp, 4 in. long x ½ in.	2 (⅔ oz)
English muffin	½
Hot dog or hamburger bun	½ (1 oz)
Pita, 6 in. across	½
Raisin bread, unfrosted	1 slice (1 oz)
Roll, plain, small	1 (1oz)
Tortilla, corn, 6 in. across	1
Tortilla, flour, 6 in. across	1
Waffle, 4½ in. square, reduced-fat	1

CEREALS AND GRAINS

Bran cereals	½ cup
Bulgur	½ cup
Cereals	½ cup
Cereals, unsweetened, ready-to-eat	¾ cup
Cornmeal (dry)	3 Tbsp.

Couscous . . . . ⅓ cup
Flour (dry) . . . . .3 Tbsp.
Granola, low-fat . . . . .¼ cup
Grape-Nuts® . . . . .¼ cup
Grits . . . . .½ cup
Kasha . . . . .½ cup
Millet . . . . .¼ cup
Muesli . . . . .¼ cup
Oats . . . . .½ cup
Pasta . . . . .½ cup
Puffed cereal . . . . .1½ cups
Rice milk . . . . .½ cup
Rice, white or brown . . . . ⅓ cup
Shredded Wheat® . . . . .½ cup
Sugar-frosted cereal . . . . .½ cup
Wheat germ . . . . .3 Tbsp

STARCHY VEGETABLES

Baked beans . . . . ⅓ cup
Corn . . . . .½ cup
Corn on cob, medium . . . . .1 (5 oz)
Mixed vegetables with corn, peas, or pasta . . . . .1 cup
Peas, green . . . . .½ cup
Plantain . . . . .½ cup
Potato, baked or boiled . . . . .1 small (3 oz)
Potato, mashed . . . . .½ cup
Squash, winter (acorn, butternut) . . . . .1 cup
Yam, sweet potato, plain . . . . .½ cup

CRACKERS AND SNACKS

Animal crackers 8
Graham crackers, 2½ in. square 3
Matzoh . . . . .¾ oz
Melba toast . . . . .4 slices
Oyster crackers 24
Popcorn (popped, no fat added or low-fat microwave) 3 cups
Pretzels . . . . .¾ oz

Rice cakes, 4 in. across 2
Saltine-type crackers 6
Snack chips, fat-free (tortilla, potato) . . . . . . .15–20 (¾ oz)
Whole-wheat crackers, no fat added . . . . .2–5 (¾ oz)

BEANS, PEAS, AND LENTILS
(Count as 1 starch exchange, plus 1 very lean meat exchange.)
Beans and peas (garbanzo, pinto,
    kidney, white, split, black-eyed) . . . . .½ cup
Lima beans . . . . .⅔ cup
Lentils . . . . .½ cup
Miso* . . . . .3 Tbsp
                * = 400 mg or more of sodium per exchange.

STARCHY FOODS, PREPARED WITH FAT
(Count as 1 starch exchange, plus 1 fat exchange.)
Biscuit, 2½ in. across 1
Chow mein noodles . . . . .½ cup
Corn bread, 2 in. cube .1 (2 oz)
Crackers, round butter type 6
Croutons . . . . .1 cup
French-fried potatoes . . . . .16–25 (3 oz)
Granola . . . . .¼ cup
Muffin, small . . . . .1 (1½ oz)
Pancake, 4 in. across 2
Popcorn, microwave . . . . .3 cups
Sandwich crackers, cheese or peanut butter filling 3
Stuffing, bread (prepared) .⅓ cup
Taco shell, 6 in. across 2
Waffle, 4½ in. square 1
Whole-wheat crackers, fat added . . . . .4–6 (1 oz)

Starches often swell in cooking, so a small amount of uncooked starch will become a much larger amount of cooked food. The following table shows some of the changes.

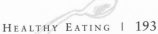

Food (Starch Group)	Uncooked	Cooked
Oatmeal	3 Tbsp	½ cup
Cream of Wheat	2 Tbsp	½ cup
Grits	3 Tbsp	½ cup
Rice	2 Tbsp	⅓ cup
Spaghetti	¼ cup	½ cup
Noodles	⅓ cup	½ cup
Macaroni	¼ cup	½ cup
Dried beans	¼ cup	½ cup
Dried peas	¼ cup	½ cup
Lentils	3 Tbsp	½ cup

Common Measurements

3 tsp = 1 Tbsp

4 Tbsp = ¼ cup

5⅓ Tbsp = ⅓ cup

4 ounces = ½ cup

8 ounces = 1 cup

1 cup = ½ pint

LIST 2: FRUIT EXCHANGES

Fresh, frozen, canned, and dried fruits and fruit juices are on this list. In general, one fruit exchange is:
• 1 small to medium fresh fruit,
• ½ cup of canned or fresh fruit or fruit juice,
• ¼ cup of dried fruit.

One fruit exchange equals:
• 15 grams carbohydrate and
• 60 calories.
• The weight includes skin, core, seeds, and rind.

FRUIT

Apple, unpeeled, small . . . . .1 (4 oz)

Applesauce, unsweetened .½ cup

Apples, dried . . . . .4 rings

Apricots, fresh . . . . .4 whole (5½ oz)

Apricots, dried . . . . .8 halves

Apricots, canned . . . . .½ cup

Banana, small . . . . .1 (4 oz)

Blackberries . . . . .¾ cup

Blueberries . . . . .¾ cup

Cantaloupe, small . . . . . . .⅓ melon (11 oz) or 1 cup cubes

Cherries, sweet, fresh . . . . .12 (3 oz)

Cherries, sweet, canned .½ cup

Dates 3

Figs, fresh . . . . .1½ large or 2 medium (3½ oz)

Figs, dried 1½

Fruit cocktail . . . . .½ cup

Grapefruit, large . . . . .½ (11 oz)

Grapefruit sections, canned . . . . .¾ cup

Grapes, small . . . . .17 (3 oz)

Honeydew melon . . . . .1 slice (10 oz) or 1 cup cubes

Kiwi . . . . .1 (3½ oz)

Mandarin oranges, canned . . . . .¾ cup

Mango, small . . . . .½ fruit (5½ oz) or ½ cup

Nectarine, small . . . . .1 (5 oz)

Orange, small . . . . .1 (6½ oz)

Papaya . . . . .½ fruit (8 oz) or 1 cup cubes

Peach, medium, fresh . . . . .1 (6 oz)

Peaches, canned . . . . .½ cup

Pear, large, fresh . . . . .½ (4 oz)

Pears, canned . . . . .½ cup

Pineapple, fresh . . . . .¾ cup

Pineapple, canned . . . . .½ cup

Plums, small . . . . .2 (5 oz)

Plums, canned . . . . .½ cup

Prunes, dried 3

Raisins . . . . .2 Tbsp

Raspberries . . . . .1 cup

Strawberries . . . . .1¼ cup whole berries
Tangerines, small . . . . .2 (8 oz)
Watermelon . . . . .1 slice (13½ oz) or 1¼ cup cubes

FRUIT JUICE
Apple juice/cider . . . . .½ cup
Cranberry juice cocktail . . . . .⅓ cup
Cranberry juice cocktail, reduced-calorie . . . . .1 cup
Fruit juice blends, 100% juice . . . . .⅓ cup
Grape juice . . . . .⅓ cup
Grapefruit juice . . . . .½ cup
Orange juice . . . . .½ cup
Pineapple juice . . . . .½ cup
Prune juice . . . . .⅓ cup

List 3: Milk Exchanges

One milk exchange equals:
- 12 grams carbohydrate and
- 8 grams protein.

SKIM AND LOW-FAT MILK
(0–3 grams fat per serving)
Skim milk . . . . .1 cup
½ % milk . . . . .1 cup
1% milk . . . . .1 cup
Nonfat or low-fat buttermilk . . . . .1 cup
Evaporated skim milk . . . . .½ cup
Nonfat dry milk . . . . .⅓ cup dry
Plain nonfat yogurt . . . . .¾ cup
Nonfat or low-fat fruit-flavored yogurt sweetened
   with aspartame or with a non-nutritive sweetener . . .1 cup

REDUCED-FAT
(5 grams fat per serving)
2% milk . . . . .1 cup
Plain low-fat yogurt . . . . .¾ cup
Sweet acidophilus milk . . . . .1 cup

WHOLE MILK

(8 grams fat per serving)

Whole milk . . . . .1 cup

Evaporated whole milk . . . . .½ cup

Goat's milk . . . . .1 cup

Kefir . . . . .1 cup

LIST 4: VEGETABLE EXCHANGES

In general, one vegetable exchange is:
- ½ cup of cooked vegetables or vegetable juice,
- 1 cup of raw vegetables.

One vegetable exchange equals:
- 5 grams carbohydrate,
- 2 grams protein,
- 0 grams fat, and
- 25 calories.

Artichoke
Artichoke hearts
Asparagus
Beans (green, wax, Italian)
Bean sprouts
Beets
Broccoli
Brussels sprouts
Cabbage
Carrots
Cauliflower
Celery
Cucumber
Eggplant
Green onions or scallions
Greens (collard, kale, mustard, turnip)
Kohlrabi
Leeks

Mixed vegetables (without corn, peas, or pasta)
Mushrooms
Okra
Onions
Pea pods
Peppers (all varieties)
Radishes
Salad greens (endive, escarole, lettuce, romaine, spinach)
Sauerkraut*
Spinach
Summer squash
Tomato
Tomatoes, canned
Tomato sauce*
Tomato/vegetable juice*

Turnips	Watercress
Water chestnuts	Zucchini

* = 400 mg or more sodium per exchange

LIST 5: MEAT EXCHANGES

In general, one meat exchange is:
- 1 oz meat, fish, poultry, or cheese,
- ½ cup beans, peas, or lentils.

Very-Lean Meat And Substitutes List
One exchange equals:
- 0 grams carbohydrate,
- 7 grams protein,
- 0–1 grams fat, and
- 35 calories.

One very-lean meat exchange is equal to any one of the following items.

POULTRY: Chicken or turkey (white meat, no skin),
 Cornish hen (no skin) . . . . .1 oz
FISH: Fresh or frozen cod, flounder, haddock, halibut,
 trout; tuna fresh or canned in water . . . . .1 oz
SHELLFISH: Clams, crab, lobster, scallops, shrimp,
 imitation shellfish . . . . .1 oz
GAME: Duck or pheasant (no skin), venison,
 buffalo, ostrich . . . . .1 oz
CHEESE with 1 gram or less fat per ounce:
 Nonfat or low-fat cottage cheese . . . . .¼ cup
 Fat-free cheese . . . . .1 oz
OTHER: Processed sandwich meats with 1 gram or less
 fat per ounce, such as deli thin, shaved meats,
 chipped beef*, turkey ham . . . . .1 oz
 Egg whites 2
 Egg substitutes, plain . . . . .¼ cup

Hot dogs with 1 gram or less fat per ounce* . . . . .1 oz
Kidney (high in cholesterol) . . . . .1 oz
Sausage with 1 gram or less fat per ounce . . . . . . .1 oz

Count as one very lean meat and one starch exchange.
Beans, peas, lentils (cooked) . . . . .½ cup
* = 400 mg or more sodium per exchange.

LEAN MEAT AND SUBSTITUTES LIST
One exchange equals:
- 0 grams carbohydrate,
- 7 grams protein,
- 3 grams fat, and
- 55 calories.

One lean meat exchange is equal to any one of the following items:

BEEF: USDA Select or Choice grades of lean beef
     trimmed of fat, such as round, sirloin, and flank
     steak; tenderloin; roast (rib, chuck, rump); steak
     (T-bone, porterhouse, cubed), ground round . . . . . .1 oz
PORK: Lean pork, such as fresh ham; canned, cured,
     or boiled ham; Canadian bacon*; tenderloin, center
     loin chop . . . . .1 oz
     Lamb: Roast, chop, leg . . . . .1 oz
VEAL: Lean chop, roast . . . . .1 oz
POULTRY: Chicken, turkey (dark meat, no skin),
     chicken (white meat, with skin), domestic
     duck or goose (well-drained of fat, no skin) . . . . . . .1 oz
FISH: Herring (uncreamed or smoked) . . . . .1 oz
     Oysters . . . . .6 medium
     Salmon (fresh or canned), catfish . . . . .1 oz
     Sardines (canned) .2 medium
     Tuna (canned in oil, drained) . . . . .1 oz
GAME: Goose (no skin), rabbit . . . . .1 oz
CHEESE: 4.5%-fat cottage cheese . . . . ¼ cup

Grated Parmesan . . . . .2 Tbsp
Cheese with 3 grams or less fat per ounce . . . . . . .1 oz
OTHER:
Hot dogs with 3 grams or less fat per ounce* . . .1½ oz
Processed sandwich meat with 3 grams or less
fat per ounce, such as turkey pastrami or kielbasa . .1 oz
Liver, heart (high in cholesterol) . . . . .1 oz
* = 400 mg or more sodium per exchange.

MEDIUM-FAT MEAT AND SUBSTITUTES LIST
One exchange equals:
- 0 grams carbohydrate,
- 7 grams protein,
- 5 grams fat, and
- 75 calories.

One medium-fat meat exchange is equal to any one of the
following items.
BEEF: Most beef products fall into this category (ground
beef, meatloaf, corned beef, short ribs, prime
grades of meat trimmed of fat, such as prime rib) . .1 oz
PORK: Top loin, chop, Boston butt, cutlet . . . . .1 oz
LAMB: Rib roast, ground . . . . .1 oz
VEAL: Cutlet (ground or cubed, unbreaded) . . . . .1 oz
POULTRY: Chicken (dark meat, with skin), ground turkey
or ground chicken, fried chicken (with skin) . . . . . . .1 oz
FISH: Any fried fish product . . . . .1 oz
CHEESE: With 5 grams or less fat per ounce
Feta . . . . .1 oz
Mozzarella . . . . .1 oz
Ricotta . . . . .¼ cup (2 oz)
OTHER:
Egg (high in cholesterol, limit to 3 per week) 1
Sausage with 5 grams or less fat per ounce . . . . . .1 oz
Soy milk . . . . .1 cup
Tempeh . . . . .¼ cup
Tofu . . . . .4 oz or ½ cup

LIST 6: FAT EXCHANGES

Fats are divided into three groups, based on the main type of fat they contain: monounsaturated, polyunsaturated, and saturated. Saturated fats are linked with heart disease and cancer, and saturated fats have been associated with an *increase* in blood cholesterol (a possible risk factor in coronary heart disease). A physician may advise a reduction of foods high in this kind of fat. If you are going to add fats, it's best to pick fats from the monounsaturated fats list. In general, one fat exchange is:

- 1 teaspoon of regular margarine or vegetable oil, or
- 1 tablespoon of regular salad dressing.

MONOUNSATURATED FATS LIST
One fat exchange equals 5 grams fat and 45 calories.

Avocado, medium	⅛ (1 oz)
Oil (canola, olive, peanut)	1 tsp
Olives: ripe (black)	8 large
green, stuffed*	10 large
Nuts: almonds, cashews	6 nuts
mixed (50% peanuts)	6 nuts
peanuts	10 nuts
pecans	4 halves
Peanut butter, smooth or crunchy	2 tsp
Sesame seeds	1 Tbsp
Tahini paste	2 tsp

POLYUNSATURATED FATS LIST
One fat exchange equals 5 grams fat and 45 calories.

Margarine: stick, tub, or squeeze	1 tsp
lower-fat (30% to 50% vegetable oil)	1 Tbsp
Mayonnaise: regular	1 tsp
reduced-fat	1 Tbsp
Nuts, walnuts, English	4 halves

```
Oil (corn, safflower, soybean) . . . . . . . . . . . . . . . . . .1 tsp
Salad dressing: regular* . . . . . . . . . . . . . . . . . . . . . . .1 Tbsp
        reduced-fat . . . . . . . . . . . . . . . . . . . . . . . . . . . .2 Tbsp
Miracle Whip®: regular . . . . . . . . . . . . . . . . . . . . . . .2 tsp
        reduced-fat . . . . . . . . . . . . . . . . . . . . . . . . . . . .1 Tbsp
Seeds: pumpkin, sunflower . . . . . . . . . . . . . . . . . .1 Tbsp
```
                                    * = 400 mg or more sodium per exchange

SATURATED FATS LIST **

One fat exchange equals 5 grams of fat and 45 calories.

```
Bacon, cooked . . . . . . . . . . . . . . . . . . . .1 slice (20 slices/lb)
Bacon, grease . . . . . . . . . . . . . . . . . . . . . . . . . . . . . .1 tsp
Butter: stick . . . . . . . . . . . . . . . . . . . . . . . . . . . . . . .1 tsp
        whipped . . . . . . . . . . . . . . . . . . . . . . . . . . . . .2 tsp
        reduced-fat . . . . . . . . . . . . . . . . . . . . . . . . . . .1 Tbsp
Chitterlings, boiled . . . . . . . . . . . . . . . . . . . .1 Tbsp (½ oz)
Coconut, sweetened, shredded . . . . . . . . . . . . . . .2 Tbsp
Cream, half and half . . . . . . . . . . . . . . . . . . . . . . . .2 Tbsp
Cream cheese: regular . . . . . . . . . . . . . . . .1 Tbsp (½ oz)
        reduced-fat . . . . . . . . . . . . . . . . . . . .2 Tbsp (1 oz)
Fatback or salt pork, see below
Shortening or lard . . . . . . . . . . . . . . . . . . . . . . . . . .1 tsp
Sour cream: regular . . . . . . . . . . . . . . . . . . . . . . . .2 Tbsp
        reduced-fat . . . . . . . . . . . . . . . . . . . . . . . . . . .3 Tbsp
```

Use a piece 1 in. x 1 in. x 1¼ in. if you plan to eat the fatback cooked with vegetables. Use a piece 2 in. x 1 in. x ½ in. when eating only the vegetables with the fatback removed.

                    ** Saturated fats can raise blood cholesterol levels.

FREE FOODS LIST

Foods with a serving size listed should be limited to three servings per day maximum. Many fat-free foods are high in sugar and may have trace amounts of fats that can add extra calories.

FAT-FREE OR REDUCED-FAT FOODS

Cream cheese, fat-free . . . . .1 Tbsp

Creamers, nondairy, liquid . . . . .1 Tbsp

Creamers, nondairy, powdered . . . . .2 tsp

Mayonnaise, fat-free . . . . .1 Tbsp

Mayonnaise, reduced-fat .1 tsp

Margarine, fat-free . . . . .4 Tbsp

Margarine, reduced-fat . . . . .1 tsp

Miracle Whip®, non-fat . . . . .1 Tbsp

Miracle Whip®, reduced-fat . . . . .1 tsp

Nonstick cooking spray

Salad dressing, fat-free . . . . .1 Tbsp

Salad dressing, fat-free, Italian . . . . .1 Tbsp

Salsa . . . . .¼ cup

Sour cream, fat-free, reduced-fat . . . . .1 Tbsp

Whipped topping, regular or light . . . . 2 Tbsp

SUGAR-FREE OR LOW-SUGAR FOODS

Candy, hard, sugar-free . . . . .1 candy

Gelatin dessert, sugar-free

Gelatin, unflavored

Gum, sugar-free

Jam or jelly, low-sugar or light . . . . 2 tsp

Sugar substitutes

Syrup, sugar-free . . . . .2 Tbsp

Sugar substitutes, alternatives, or replacements that are approved by the Food and Drug Administration (FDA) are safe to use. Common brand names include:

Equal® (aspartame)

Sprinkle Sweet® (saccharin)

Sweet One® (acesulfame K)

Sweet-10® (saccharin)

Sugar Twin® (saccharin)

Sweet 'n Low® (saccharin)

DRINKS
Bouillon, broth, consommé*
Bouillon or broth, low-sodium
Carbonated or mineral water
Club soda
Cocoa powder, unsweetened . . . . .1 Tbsp
Coffee
Diet soft drinks, sugar-free
Drink mixes, sugar-free
Tea
Tonic water, sugar-free

CONDIMENTS
Catsup . . . . .1 Tbsp
Horseradish
Lemon juice
Limejuice
Mustard
Pickles, dill* . . . . .1½ large
Soy sauce, regular or light *
Taco sauce . . . . .1 Tbsp
Vinegar

SEASONINGS
Be careful with seasonings that contain sodium or are salts,
such as garlic or celery salt, and lemon pepper.
Flavoring extracts
Garlic
Herbs, fresh or dried
Pimento
Spices
Tabasco® or hot pepper sauce
Wine, used in cooking
Worcestershire sauce

                    * = 400 mg or more of sodium per exchange.

How much fat?

The latest recommendation from the American Institute for Cancer Research recommends that total fat intake should be between 15% to no more than 30% of a person's total daily calories. This is in keeping with the American Heart Association's Guidelines to help reduce high cholesterol and heart disease.

Below is a fat budget plan showing you different fat gram amounts for different calorie levels. One is worked out for 25% fat calories, the second for 20%, and the third for 15%. Now here is the really hard part: you should not go any lower than the lowest figure on this chart for your daily calorie allowance. Fat is essential in your diet to maintain normal metabolism—too little fat is not good. After looking over the chart, pray and decide what you should do for the next 12 weeks—and fill in the sentence at the bottom of the page with your commitment.

If you follow the meal plans (see pg. 226) and choose primarily non-fat dairy products and extra lean or lean meats from the exchange lists, you will easily be within the recommended range. You may want to take the time to actually add up the fat grams you ate for a few days so you can double check that you are meeting your fat gram goals.

FAT BUDGET PLAN

Daily Caloric Allowance	1000	1200	1500	1850	2000	2400
25% Fat Calories (Daily calories x .25)	250	300	375	463	500	600
# Fat Grams allowed (Fat calories ÷ 9)	28	33	41	51	55	67
Daily Caloric Allowance	1000	1200	1500	1850	2000	2400
20% Fat Calories (Daily calories x .2)	200	240	300	370	400	480
# Fat Grams allowed (Fat calories ÷ 9)	22	26	33	41	44	53
Daily Caloric Allowance	1000	1200	1500	1850	2000	2400
15% Fat Calories (Daily calories x .15)	150	180	225	278	300	360
# Fat Grams allowed (Fat calories ÷ 9)	17	20	25	31	33	40

My Personal Fat Budget should be _____ grams of fat for the first 12 weeks of 3D. It is _____% of _____ calories daily.

LET'S NOT FORGET THE FIBER

Most experts recommend that people eat between 20 and 30 grams of fiber daily. Most of us eat less than 12 grams. Some simple ways to boost your fiber intake are:

1. Choose *whole-grain* bread and bread products.
2. Start your day with a high-fiber cereal.
3. Instead of white rice or pasta, try wild rice or whole wheat couscous for an exciting new side dish.
4. Add a serving of beans or lentils to your usual menu.
5. Keep a supply of cut-up fruits and vegetables handy for snacking.

Look at the list below to get an idea of high-fiber foods.

High-Fiber Foods

Grains	Grams Fiber
Popcorn (3 c)	2.7
Bread (1 sl)	
Whole Wheat	1.6
White	0.5
Rice (1 c)	
Brown	3.3
White	1.0
Bulgur (1 c)	7.8
Barley (1 c)	6.5
Couscous (1 c)	21
Whole Wheat	
Couscous (1 c cooked)	7

Cereals (1 oz)	Grams Fiber*
Fiber One® (½ c)	14.0
All-Bran® (½ c)	10.0
Bran Flakes (¾ c)	5.0
Multi-Bran Chex® (¾ c)	4.0
Wheat Chex® (¾ c)	5.0
Quaker Corn Bran (¾ c)	5.0
Raisin Bran (½ c)	
Post	4.5
Kellogg's®	3.5
Fruit and Fibre® (½ c)	4.0
Oat Bran	
Cooked (⅔ c)	5.0
Shredded Wheat (1)	3.0
Total (¾ c)	2.5
Wheaties® (1 c)	3.0
Wheat Germ (3 tbsp)	3.3
Oatmeal, cooked	
Regular (½ c)	4.0
Multi-Grain (½ c)	5.0
Grape-Nuts® (¼ c)	2.5

Fruits	Grams Fiber
Apple (with skin)	2.8
Banana	3.0
Blueberries (½ c)	1.5
Orange	2.6
Pear (with skin)	4.0
Prunes (3)	1.6
Strawberries (1 c)	3.9

Crackers (½ oz)	Grams Fiber*
Wasa Crispbread	
Fiber Plus (1½)	4.3
Sesame Rye (1½)	3.6
Ryvita Crispbread	
High Fiber (1½)	2.5
Kavli Crispbread	
Thick (1½)	3.0
Ry-Krisp Natural or	
Seasoned (2 triples)	3.0

Legumes	Grams Fiber
(½ cup cooked)	
Black Beans	6.5
Kidney Beans	5.0
Pinto Beans	5.9
Chick-peas	4.4
Lentils	7.8
Lima Beans	4.0

Starchy Vegetables	Grams Fiber
(½ cup cooked)	
Peas	3.0
Corn	3.4
Potato, baked	1.6
Squash, summer	1.5
Squash, winter	3.0
Yams	3.8

Vegetables	Grams Fiber
(1 cup raw)	
Broccoli	2.2
Cabbage	1.5
Carrots	4.6
Green Beans	3.5
Lettuce	0.5
Spinach	1.5
Tomatoes	2.4
Asparagus	2.5

The Food Guide Pyramid from the USDA has become widely recognized as an educational tool for dietary assessment. It visually illustrates what to eat each day. It is not a rigid plan, but a guide that shows you how to choose a healthful diet. The Food Guide Pyramid emphasizes foods from the five food groups, in the lower three sections. This is just a basic guide, not specific for individual needs such as lactose intolerance, or for African, Asian, Hispanic, or Native American eating habits. Others have adapted this guide to their needs. We hope this will help you, too.

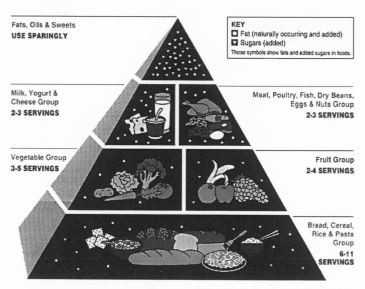

Courtesy of the U.S. Department of Agriculture

Nutritional Notes

PROTEINS are the body's building blocks; you need them for muscle and connective tissue growth. They do not stimulate your body's insulin production, and that means your blood sugar doesn't drop and you don't feel as hungry later on. Proteins also take a little while to digest, so they make you feel fuller longer. Too much protein or any one nutrient is not good for your body. Avoid diets that are extreme in any one nutrient. Think balance!

CARBOHYDRATES supply vital nutritional needs in our diet and are our primary source of fuel. Carbohydrates can be found in many food sources including milk, grains, fruits, and vegetables. Items like sugar, honey, molasses, and corn syrup are primarily pure carbohydrates and are often called simple sugars because of their molecular structure. Unlike protein, when you ingest carbohydrates, your blood sugar rises. Food made from simple carbohydrates, like candy bars, cookies, and soft drinks, can cause a rapid rise in your blood sugar level. This rapid rise can cause a stimulatory effect, which is often why people turn to sweets for a "pick-up" or energy boost. After the rapid rise, a fall in blood sugar usually occurs and the person may crave more sweets. This is how a cycle of eating too many sweets and overeating begins.

Carbohydrates can also be classified according to whether they contain whole grains or refined. The refined carbohydrates, such as refined white bread, lower good HDL cholesterol—something you don't want to do. Meanwhile, the whole grains, including brown rice, oats, and whole-wheat pasta, metabolize more slowly, providing a beneficial effect.

Some people are more carbohydrate sensitive than others. If you know you have difficulty handling your sweet intake, it's best to always avoid dessert food. It is also important that your total daily carbohydrate is not in excess. Remember to keep your meals balanced and to eat regular snacks. These strategies, which form part of the 3D program, will help minimize cravings for sweets and will help you stay energetic throughout the day.

FATS increase the viscosity (stickiness) of blood, and sticky blood clumps together and attaches to the walls of blood vessels, interfering with blood flow and cell breathing. A lot is being written about the danger of high-fat diets. They can increase your risk of a stroke or heart attack and have also been implicated in certain cancers, particularly of the bowel and breast. You will ingest fat in many of the foods you eat normally, so it is best to avoid increasing your fat intake if at all possible. Triglycerides are fats normally present in the blood that are made from food. Being overweight or consuming too much fat, alcohol, and sugar may increase the blood triglycerides to an unacceptably high level.

Therefore, we recommend eating more good fats (polyunsaturated and monounsaturated)—such as those found in olive, canola, or peanut oil, as well as in fish—and less of the saturated fats.

CHOLESTEROL is a fatty substance produced by our bodies that is an essential part of every cell. Cholesterol is also found in foods of animal origin—eggs, milk, meat, fish, and poultry. Too much dietary cholesterol is unnecessary and may be harmful.

Too much cholesterol is harmful because saturated fat and dietary cholesterol (cholesterol in your food) are contributors to increased levels of total blood cholesterol in your body. Increased levels of total blood cholesterol have been identified as a risk factor for atherosclerosis—a build-up of fatty deposits on the inner walls of the blood vessels. Atherosclerosis is a leading risk factor for heart disease and stroke.

There are different kinds of cholesterol. Cholesterol is one blood reading that has several parts. The LDL-Cholesterol (low-density lipoprotein) and the HDL-Cholesterol (high-density lipoprotein) make up your blood cholesterol. The LDL-Cholesterol is the most harmful.

LDL is commonly known as the "bad" cholesterol because it deposits artery-clogging cholesterol on the walls of the blood vessels. HDL, on the other hand, is called the "good" cholesterol, because it sweeps cholesterol out of the body.

Cholesterol is measured by a simple blood test that shows milligrams of total cholesterol (HDL and LDL) per deciliter of blood. Total cholesterol over 185 mg/dl for children or 240mg/dl for adults is undesirably high.

The American Heart Association recommends that healthy adults eat no more than 300mg of dietary cholesterol per day. By eating fewer animal products and saturated fats, and eating more fruits, vegetables, fish, and whole grains, you can reduce your dietary cholesterol. Choose polyunsaturated and monounsaturated fat rather than saturated fat.

(National Institute of Health)

The 8 best cooking oils have the least saturated fat and no cholesterol:

Canola	Peanut
Safflower	Olive
Sunflower	Soybean
Corn	Rice Bran

Here are 6 fats to avoid; although they are choles-terol-free, their high saturated fat levels will raise blood cholesterol:

Vegetable Shortening	Palm Oil
Cottonseed Oil	Lard
Animal Fat Shortening	Coconut

All of these fats need to be considered in your FAT exchanges. Even though the label says "No Cholesterol," they are all 100 percent fat—45 calories per teaspoon.

FIBER—An indigestible part of certain foods. Fiber is important in the diet as roughage, or bulk. Fiber is found in foods from the starch/bread, vegetable, and fruit exchange lists.

SOLUBLE FIBER has high water-holding capability and turns to gel during digestion. This process slows diges-tion and the rate of nutrient absorption from the stom-ach and intestine. Soluble fiber is found in oat bran, pectin (from fruits and vegetables), and various "gums" which are found in nuts, seeds, and legumes such as beans, lentils, and peas. This type of fiber may play a role in smoothing out the glycemic response of foods, and in reducing the likelihood of atherosclerosis.

INSOLUBLE FIBER is found in foods such as wheat bran and other whole grains, and has poor water-holding capability. It appears to speed the passage of foods through the stomach and intestines, and increases fecal bulk. This type of fiber probably does not affect glycemic response or atherosclerosis.

USE LESS SALT—Most of us eat too much salt. The sodium in salt can cause the body to retain water, and in some people it may raise blood pressure. High blood pressure is made worse by eating too much salt and sodium. So try to use less salt in cooking and at the table. Decrease the amount of high-sodium foods such as ham, bacon, salted crackers, pickles, olives, and canned soups.

Hints

As you proceed through the twelve-week 3D session, you might crave some special favorite foods—particularly at holiday times. Try to fix these foods and their ingredients into the Exchange Lists and still remain on the diet.

Read labels. Low-calorie, reduced calorie or lite does not mean calorie-free. This is especially true of "low-calorie" salad dressings, some of which contain up to 40 or 50 calories per tablespoon. We advise using only those that have fewer than ten calories per tablespoon. The word "dietetic" can be misleading; it, too, does not mean calorie-free, and even products labeled "dietetic" should not be eaten in large amounts—an overall balance is healthy.

Keep non-fat dry milk and skimmed evaporated milk on hand. These are easy to cook with and have fewer calories than modified skimmed milk.

Buy natural fruit juices. Imitation fruit juices contain very little fruit juice and do contain much sugar and many calories.

Learn about spices and condiments; many add flavor but not calories. You can use herbs and spices, rather than butter, to season vegetables. Spices can be used in sauces and salad dressings, in soups, stews, and meat loaf, and in fish, beef and poultry dishes. Dry mustard, garlic powder and garlic salt, onion powder and onion salt, celery seed and salt, curry powder, paprika, and dill seed are some of the spices and herbs that can be used in daily cooking. Did you know that paprika has more Vitamin C than any of the citrus fruits? Be bold in experimenting, using very small amounts to "test the taste," and you will soon discover your own favorites.

For a taste treat, try adding a bit of cinnamon, allspice, nutmeg, ginger, mace, or cloves to quick breads or muffins or coffee cakes, or to custards and creams, or add to root vegetables or the fall squashes for a different, delightful flavor.

The difference between salad and steamed vegetables is that steaming ruptures the starch molecule and makes for more satisfying food than just the bulk and fiber of salad. If the vegetables are steamed lightly, they will retain the filling quality of fiber and still unlock the starch.

When it is difficult to weigh food there is a way to "eye-ball" amounts. One ounce of meat is the size of a small matchbox, 3 ounces of meat is the size of a deck of cards, and 8 ounces of meat is the size of a small paperback book.

In restaurants you can substitute fruit for the normal first courses.

Drink eight glasses of water daily.

Vegetarian Diet

We frequently receive inquiries regarding a Vegetarian Diet Plan. To meet that request, we have included an explanation of the Vegetarian Diet and a Model Diet Pattern Chart indicating calories and exchanges.

Pure vegetarians do not eat any foods of any animal origin for health reasons. Vegetarianism is gaining in popularity as many find that even occasional vegetarian meals help in lowering both food costs and fat consumption, and contribute fiber to the diet.

Lacto-ovo vegetarians who use eggs and dairy products as well as a variety of peas, beans, lentils, seeds, and nuts have no difficulty getting enough protein.

Vegans, who eliminate all animal products from their menus, must plan their meals more carefully. They will need serving sizes large enough to meet protein needs because plant proteins are less digestible than animal proteins. Vegans also need to plan their meals around complementary protein combinations. Because a vegan meal is bulky and low in protein digestibility, infants and young children will have difficulty eating enough of the plant protein choices to meet their recommended daily intakes for protein and iron. Vegans choose this diet primarily for philosophical reasons rather than health reasons.

In recent years, our affluent society has allowed most Americans to include meat in their diet. Lately, with the rising cost of meat and the latest medical findings that indicate a need to decrease dietary cholesterol and fats, many Americans are trying to cut down on their meat intake. The U.S. Recommended Dietary Allowance for protein has been *decreased* from 70 to 56 grams per day for men and from 55 to

46 grams for women, indicating that we do not need as much meat as we have been used to in the past.

How then do you plan a meatless diet and still eat the necessary protein and vitamins? While we may not need as much protein as we thought, we *do* need high-quality protein—that is, protein that has the essential amino acids. Proteins are the basis for all living tissue. There is no living tissue that does not contain some protein. The animal eats protein, whether animal or vegetable, breaks it down into amino acids by digestion, absorbs the amino acids, and from them forms its own protein. Therefore the amino acids are the units or the building stones from which the complex structure, protein, is built.

Experiments have been done which indicate that some amino acids are far more valuable than others. Animal proteins are, in general, well balanced in their amino acid distribution, whereas the protein in vegetables often is not complete in itself. When you learn how to *combine the various vegetables* you can form complete protein containing the proper amino acids. Although it is not our intent to give a complete course on combining foods, we do want to communicate how simple it is to combine the various vegetable proteins to obtain a complete protein such as is found in meat.

To achieve the right balance of vegetable proteins, it is important to choose a variety of fruits and vegetables. The dark green, leafy vegetables such as collards, kale, spinach, turnip and mustard greens, supply calcium and riboflavin; cabbage and broccoli also contain some calcium. Dried fruits, whole grains, and green leafy vegetables are also good sources of iron. Legumes, nuts and other seeds are good sources of the B-vitamins, along with germ and bran cereal grains. When a plant, or a portion of a plant, is rich in vitamins, it is also rich in minerals. So there is a variety of vitamins and minerals in fruits, green leafy vegetables, whole grains, legumes and other seeds and nuts.

The cereal grains comprise another important group, especially in their unrefined form. It has been found that the protein in the whole grain is a superior product in quality and quantity, and the best protein is found in the germ and the bran. Whole-grain cereals and bread provide a moderate amount of protein, B-vitamins and minerals, but it is when the cereal grains are *combined* in a meal with legumes, such as peas and beans, that a complete protein is formed.

Legumes are a large group of plants of the pea family, having pods containing seeds. They have a higher protein content than any other vegetable family and they also enrich the soil with nitrogen.

In summary, here are some suggested combinations for complementary protein menu ideas:

1. Rice and beans
2. Wheat-soy bread
3. Baked beans and whole wheat bread
4. Pea soup and corn bread
5. Corn tortillas and beans
6. Whole-wheat bread and milk or cheese
7. Pasta with milk or cheese
8. Rice and milk pudding

COMPLEMENTARY PLANT PROTEIN SOURCES

Food	Complementary Protein
Grains	Rice + legumes
	Corn + legumes
	Wheat + legumes
	Wheat + peanuts + milk
	Wheat + sesame + soybeans
	Rice + sesame
	Rice + brewer's yeast
Legumes	Legumes + rice
	Beans + wheat
	Beans + corn
	Soybeans + rice + wheat
	Soybeans + corn + milk
	Soybeans + peanuts + sesame
	Soybeans + peanuts + wheat + rice
Nuts and Seeds	Peanuts + sesame + soybeans
	Sesame + beans
	Sesame + soybeans + wheat
	Peanuts + sunflower seeds

Now that you have a better understanding of the vegetarian diet, how can you apply this in your 3D dietary program? The following chart illustrates the exchange list meal pattern for a vegetarian diet:

	1200 Calories	1500 Calories	1800 Calories
List 1 Starch	6	8	9
List 2 Fruit	3	3	5
List 3 Milk	1 cup low-fat	2 cups	2 cups
List 4 Vegetables	4	5	5
List 5 Meat	4	5	5
List 6 Fat	4	5	6

Vegetarian Diet Pattern Chart

Exchanges	CALORIES PER DAY		
	1200	1500	1800
	Number of Exchanges		
Breakfast			
Meat	1	1	1
Bread	1	1	2
Fruit	1	1	1
Milk	½	1	1
Fat	1	1	2
Lunch			
Meat	2	2	2
Bread	2	3	3
Vegetable	2	2	2
Fruit	1	1	2
Milk	½	½	½
Fat	1	1	2
Dinner			
Meat	2	2	2
Bread	3	4	4
Vegetable	2	3	3
Fruit	1	1	2
Milk	—	½	½
Fat	1	2	2

These are some non-meat protein exchanges:

LEAN MEAT:

Dried beans and peas	½ c. = 1 protein and 1 bread
Low-fat cheese	1 oz. = 1 protein
Low-fat cottage cheese	¼ c. = 1 protein
Tofu, low-fat	4 oz. (2½" x 2¾" x 1") = 1 protein

MEDIUM FAT—OMIT ½ FAT:

Cheese—Mozzarella	1 oz. = 1 protein
Ricotta	1 oz. = 1 protein
Farmer's	1 oz. = 1 protein
Neufchatel	1 oz. = 1 protein
Parmesan	1 oz. = 1 protein
Egg (whole)	1 protein

If you have seen the word *tofu* and wondered what it is, this is a kind of soy cheese made for years in the Orient from soy flour and soy flakes. This cheese-like product is found in the fresh vegetable section of the grocery store. This protein product may be sliced, cubed, cut into chunks, ground, grated, or molded into shapes, and added to casseroles. It doesn't have much flavor in itself, but it takes on the flavor of the foods that it is mixed with.

Not only is the Vegetarian Diet economical, but also it has some other clear merits. Vegetarians increase their intake of complex carbohydrates, and through avoiding meat they decrease their intake of saturated fat. All these factors are a plus according to current dietary reports.

Food Allergy Problems

Studies have shown that eating one food repeatedly can cause our bodies to build up sensitivity to that food and produce harmful effects. If you have eating habits that lean heavily on the same food meal after meal, you might want to try rotating your food over a four-day period to see if you are overloading your body's defense system. If this is happening, your white blood corpuscles are responding to the "overload" as if they were being invaded by alien microbes and you may be unduly exhausted, or suffer from frequent headaches, sinus attacks, etc. Rotating foods could relieve the body of this artificially induced strain and permit it to function more effectively.

There are two basic ways to detect the foods to which you might be acutely sensitive, and the first is a natural outgrowth of rotating our foods. It involves limiting the intake of any one food to one meal out of 12. For instance, if you ate eggs for breakfast on Monday morning, you would not eat eggs again until Friday. Rotation makes it much easier to isolate those foods that are having adverse physical and mental effects on us.

The second way to uncover hidden food allergies is to systematically eliminate one suspect food at a time from our rotation and then re-introduce it and monitor our body and emotions for any aberrant effects. This is an old but well-proven method of discovering allergies that doctors have been successfully using for generations.

Vitamins and Minerals

Vitamins and minerals are essential for human life. They serve a variety of functions and play a crucial role in many body processes. The first vitamin was discovered at the beginning of the twentieth century. When chemists discovered how to synthesize vitamins in the 1930s, deficiency-related diseases were almost eradicated by food fortification. Since then, many discoveries have been made about how vitamins and minerals contribute to optimum health. As science has progressed, so has the market for vitamin and mineral supplements. Today, many of us are overwhelmed with information about how much of a vitamin or mineral we should have, whether or not we should take supplements, and if so what is the form best absorbed by the body. There are many questions for which scientists unfortunately still do not have answers.

It is important to realize that if we eat a well-balanced diet, most of us will get all the nutrients we need. There are some vitamins that may offer health benefits when taken in amounts higher than the recommended daily allowances. If you decide to supplement, make sure you have adequate information regarding the nutrient you are taking. Some vitamins and minerals are toxic at high levels and some may interfere with the effectiveness of certain medications. We suggest that you let your doctor be aware of any supplements you are taking. If you have questions regarding supplementation, try speaking to a registered dietitian or to a health professional.

Plateaus

A plateau is the point in your diet when you stop losing weight, even though you've been faithful to your diet plan. Every diet program includes setbacks and plateaus. You need to keep moving on, knowing that the program will work, even in the times you don't see the results. Dieters frequently get discouraged when they hit plateaus. Regardless of your faithfulness to your diet, these are to be expected.

The longer the calorie reduction lasts, the more the basal metabolic rate (rate of burning energy) slows down. Your body guards the fat, records a set-point weight, and will fight to defend that set point. As soon as your body gets over the shock of the initial water loss, it begins its fight back. It fights by lowering your basal metabolic rate so that you don't burn as much fat. Reducing your caloric intake further is not the answer. Exercise, of course, helps, but faithfulness and perseverance is necessary at these times! It helps to expect these temporary lulls—they are just part of the dieting process.

Be certain to talk about any discouragement so you won't "give up."

Anorexia Nervosa

More and more we are hearing about eating disorders that include anorexia nervosa and bulimia. The 3D program can be a help to people with these problems. Many reasons behind these problems are the same as those behind overeating—"not feeling very good about who we are, constantly trying to prove our worth, over and over again, not only to parents and peers, but, most of all, to ourselves. And no matter what we achieved, it was never enough." (Quoted from *Deadly Diet*.)

To an anorexic, being or becoming overweight is the worst thing that can happen. Fat is disgusting and repulsive, and to be fat is to be a failure. Many have painful memories of teasing and rejection as children. Being in control of their food gives anorexics a feeling of safety.

The rigid need to be perfect drives the anorexic or bulimic ruthlessly. If any goal is reached, the next goal must be higher . . . and higher. Such a person is always striving!

There is help for anorexics and bulimics if they want help. The support of a caring, sharing 3D group can be an incredible blessing. Who better than a struggling dieter (who is herself just finding new healing in the area of food) can understand another's inner agony in the area of food?

Here are a few suggestions that we believe could be helpful:

- Eat three meals a day—do not skip a meal.
- Try to eat two snacks a day also.
- Do not weigh yourself except every other week.
- Keep your food sheet honestly. If you are in a group, be sure to give your sheet to the leaders for their support and encouragement.

It is very important that you talk about your feelings. This is a terrific way to use your spiritual journal, *My Thoughts Along the Way*. How do you feel when your weight goes up? Do you feel guilty when you eat? Remember, absolutely nothing is impossible with the Lord. In fact, He specializes in impossible things. Please keep in touch with us.

Tips for Behavior Change

Try some of the following tips to help you control your food intake.

1. Rearrange food storage areas. Keep other family members' high fat/high sugar food in opaque containers (out of sight, out of mind).

2. Give away or throw away high fat/high sugar food gifts.

3. Keep healthy snacks available at work.

4. Don't eat in front of the TV set.

5. Do something enjoyable to distract yourself from eating (read a book or magazine, take a bubble bath, call a friend, find a hobby).

6. Prepare ahead. Plan and shop for meals in advance.

7. Use smaller plates and serving bowls.

8. Wait a half hour until the hunger or craving passes. Eat when you are truly hungry, not bored or stressed.

9. Choose restaurants with low-fat choices or flexible menus.

10. Reward yourself with little gifts (non-food items) for positive behavior.

Twenty-One Days of Simple, Easy-to-Plan, Low-Fat Meals

The following menus are based on exchanges for 1500 calories a day. Individuals using the 1200-calorie-a-day plan for exchanges can adjust by subtracting 1 meat, 1 bread, and 1 fruit exchange. Total fat exchanges for each day can also be adjusted by using low-fat instead of nonfat cheeses and dressings and vice versa.

The ADA recommends the following exchanges be spaced out as follows (you may, however, move those exchanges around to suit your lifestyle, and to create a snack for mid-afternoon or the evening, but be sure you get the total need for each day in each category):

Breakfast:
Meat 1
Bread 2
Fruit 1
Milk.................1

Dinner:
Meat 3
Bread 2
Vegetable........3
Fruit 1
Milk.................0
Fat...................2

Lunch:
Meat 3
Bread 2
Vegetable........2
Fruit 1
Milk.................1
Fat...................1

Totals:
Meat 7
Bread 6
Vegetable........5
Fruit 3
Milk.................2
Fat...................3

Menus

DAY 1

BREAKFAST
nonfat cottage cheese
2 pancakes
applesauce with cinnamon
4 oz skim milk

LUNCH
tuna salad with nonfat mayonnaise
2 slices whole wheat bread
celery and carrot sticks
pickles, lettuce
small banana
8 oz skim milk

DINNER
Chicken Cacciatore (recipe follows)
1 cup pasta
peaches
4 oz skim milk

DAY 2

BREAKFAST
nonfat cheese
cornflakes
berries on cereal
4 oz skim milk

LUNCH
grilled cheese sandwich
(with low-fat cheese on
rye bread)
canned non-fat tomato soup
small apple
8 oz skim milk

DINNER
stuffed baked potato with
non-fat cheese and broccoli
tossed salad with orange segments
low-fat poppy seed dressing
4 oz skim milk

DAY 3
BREAKFAST
poached egg
orange juice
4 oz skim milk
LUNCH
Polynesian Sandwich (recipe follows)
(2 servings)
pineapple
8 oz skim milk
DINNER
Baked Fish with Stuffing (recipe follows)
Romanian Vegetable Potpourri (recipe follows)
4 oz skim milk

DAY 4
BREAKFAST
nonfat cheese
Whole Wheat Raisin Bread (recipe follows), 1 slice
small apple
4 oz skim milk
LUNCH
chef salad with nonfat cheese
and lean ham
dried apricots
low-fat salad dressing
6 crackers
8 oz skim milk

DINNER
3 oz baked chicken
Corn Scallop (recipe follows)
green beans with mushrooms
fruit cocktail
4 oz skim milk

DAY 5
BREAKFAST
8 oz nonfat yogurt
Cranberry Bread (recipe follows), 1 slice
cranberry juice
4 oz skim milk
LUNCH
Healthy Choice Vegetable Soup
6 wheat crackers
Cheese sticks
small apple
8 oz skim milk
DINNER
Sloppy Joes (recipe follows)
carrots and celery sticks, pickles, lettuce
melon wedge
low-fat mayonnaise on burger
4 oz skim milk

DAY 6
BREAKFAST
nonfat cream cheese
small bagel
small banana
4 oz skim milk

Salmon Croquettes (recipe follows)
pickled beets
grapes
8 oz skim milk
DINNER
Oven Fried Chicken (recipe follows)
broccoli spears with shredded carrots
fresh pear
4 oz skim milk

DAY 7
BREAKFAST
nonfat cream cheese
2 Eggo waffles
strawberries
4 oz skim milk
LUNCH
deli turkey
small wheat tortilla
lettuce, tomato, pickles
cantaloupe wedge
low-fat mayonnaise
8 oz skim milk
DINNER
**Roasted Summer Vegetables and Chicken
(recipe follows)**
small apple
4 oz skim milk

DAY 8

BREAKFAST
nonfat cheese
shredded wheat cereal
blueberries
4 oz skim milk

LUNCH
chicken dog in roll
tomato, cucumber, lettuce
pear
nonfat dressing
8 oz skim milk

DINNER
pasta with meat sauce
tossed salad with grapefruit sections
Parmesan cheese
nonfat dressing
4 oz skim milk

DAY 9

BREAKFAST
boiled egg
2 slices whole wheat toast
orange juice
4 oz skim milk

LUNCH
Reuben Sandwich made with chicken,
sauerkraut, low-fat Swiss cheese,
and low-fat Russian dressing
2 slices rye or pumpernickel bread
apple
8 oz skim milk

Applesauce Meat Loaf (recipe follows)
baked potato
zucchini
melon wedge
4 oz skim milk

DAY 10
BREAKFAST
nonfat cream cheese
Brown Graham Bread (recipe follows)
small banana
4 oz skim milk
LUNCH
tuna salad with onion, pickle
tomato on lettuce bed
6 crackers
peach
8 oz skim milk
DINNER
Chicken with Roasted Garlic (recipe follows)
baked sweet potato
spinach
pineapple slice
4 oz skim milk

DAY 11
BREAKFAST
nonfat cream cheese
Bran Muffins (recipe follows)
blueberries
4 oz skim milk

LUNCH
Fruit medley plate
1 cup yogurt
raw veggies (cherry tomatoes,
celery and carrot sticks)
hard roll
8 oz skim milk

DINNER
Good Old Yankee Pot Roast (recipe follows)
tossed salad
nonfat dressing
baked apple
4 oz skim milk

DAY 12

BREAKFAST
1 poached egg
2 slices toast
cranberry juice
4 oz skim milk

LUNCH
grilled cheese sandwich
raw broccoli crowns
pineapple slices
8 oz skim milk

DINNER
tacos made with ground chicken or turkey
tomatoes, lettuce, salsa
low-fat cheese
nonfat sour cream
strawberries
4 oz skim milk

DAY 13

Breakfast Cobbler (recipe follows)
Blue Cheese Pear Melt
(p 744 *1001 More Low-Fat Recipes*)
tossed salad with nonfat dressing
8 oz skim milk
broiled fish
rice Pilaf
stewed tomatoes
small slice angel food cake, topped with berries
4 oz skim milk

DAY 14

2 slices toast with peanut butter
apple slices
4 oz skim milk
Shrimp Salad Sandwiches (recipe follows)
tomato slices
plum
8 oz skim milk
baked ham
German Potato Salad (recipe follows)
green beans
Apple Salad (recipe follows)
4 oz skim milk

DAY 15

BREAKFAST
Cream of Wheat cereal with shredded cheese
cranberry juice
4 oz skim milk

LUNCH
Tuna melts (recipe follows)
carrot sticks
8 oz skim milk

DINNER
Ham and Potato Casserole
(p 169 of *1001 More Low-Fat recipes*)
broccoli spears
baked apple
4 oz skim milk

DAY 16

BREAKFAST
Eggs, Southwestern Style (recipe follows)
orange juice
4 oz skim milk

LUNCH
chef salad with leftover ham
low-fat dressing
whole wheat pita bread
nectarine
8 oz skim milk

DINNER
Orange Baked Chicken (recipe follows)
yellow summer squash, zucchini halves with herbs,
grilled or broiled
wild rice
melon slices
4 oz skim milk

DAY 17

BREAKFAST
non fat cottage cheese
2 slices whole wheat toast
no-sugar jelly
1 orange
4 oz skim milk

LUNCH
hamburger from extra lean beef
English muffin
onion, tomato slices, cucumber wedges
mixed berries
8 oz skim milk

DINNER
Honey Mustard Pork Tenderloin (recipe follows)
Herb and Mushroom Rice (recipe follows)
asparagus
applesauce
4 oz skim milk

DAY 18

BREAKFAST
low-fat yogurt
dry cereal with skim milk
small banana

LUNCH
grilled cheese sandwich
canned tomato soup
lettuce wedge
nonfat dressing
small apple
8 oz skim milk

ham rollups with pickles
Best Potato Soup Ever (recipe follows)
peaches
4 oz skim milk

DAY 19

BREAKFAST
poached egg
½ English muffin
½ grapefruit
4 oz skim milk

LUNCH
Mid-Eastern Sandwiches (recipe follows)
tossed salad with non-fat dressing
8 oz skim milk

DINNER
Beef-Cabbage Casserole (recipe follows)
noodles
fruit cocktail
4 oz skim milk

DAY 20

BREAKFAST
nonfat cheese
½ English muffin
Wake-Up Shake (recipe follows)

LUNCH
nonfat cottage cheese
mixed fruit plate
6 crackers
carrots, radishes, broccoli crowns
8 oz skim milk

Easy Vegetable Soup (recipe follows)
baked apple or pear
4 oz skim milk

DAY 21

BREAKFAST
scrambled egg
2 slices whole grain toast
orange juice
4 oz skim milk

LUNCH
chicken dog in roll
onions, relish
lowfat hearty canned vegetable soup
melon wedge
8 oz skim milk

DINNER
baked fish
baked potato
Veggie Stir-Fry (recipe follows)
baked grapefruit half
4 oz skim milk

RECIPES

CHICKEN CACCIATORE

3 pounds chicken parts
¼ cup flour
½ teaspoon salt
dash pepper
⅛ cup olive oil
3 medium onions, sliced

1 green pepper, cut in strips
1 (4 oz) can mushrooms, drained
1 large clove garlic, minced
1 cup V-8 juice
½ teaspoon oregano

Combine flour, salt, and pepper.
Dust chicken with flour mixture.
In large skillet brown chicken in olive oil; remove chicken.
Brown onions and green pepper in same skillet.
Add mushrooms and garlic.
Blend in remaining ingredients.
Add chicken and cover.
Simmer about 30 minutes or until chicken is tender, stirring occasionally.
Serves 8
Exchanges = 4 extra-lean meat, ½ bread/starch, 1 vegetable

POLYNESIAN SANDWICH

1-ounce slice low-fat ham
1 slice whole grain bread
1-ounce slice low-fat cheese (Swiss, American, or your favorite)
1 slice pineapple

Butter bread on one side with ½ teaspoon butter and place on broiler. Add ham and pineapple to bread slice; place under broiler to heat through. Place cheese slice on sandwich and broil until melted.

Serves 1
Exchanges = 2 lean meat, 1 starch, 1 fruit, 1 fat

BAKED STUFFED FISH

Stuffing
¼ cup low-fat margarine
2 tablespoons chopped onion
¼ cup finely chopped celery
2 cups bread cubes
¼ teaspoon salt
¼ teaspoon dried thyme

pepper to taste

Fish
2–3 pounds dressed whole fish
½ teaspoon salt
2 tablespoons low-fat
  margarine, melted

Heat oven to 400°F. Grease a shallow roasting dish.

In medium skillet, melt ¼ cup low-fat margarine over medium heat. Add celery and onion; sauté until tender. Stir in remaining stuffing ingredients.

Sprinkle inside of fish with the ½ teaspoon of salt. Fill opening with stuffing. Secure edges of fish together with skewers or toothpicks. Place fish in greased baking dish; brush with remaining melted low-fat margarine.

Bake at 400°F for 45 minutes or until fish flakes easily with a fork, basting occasionally with low-fat margarine. Remove skewers before serving. Cut into sections to serve.

Serves 6
Exchanges = ½ starch, 5 very-lean meat, 3 fat

ROMANIAN VEGETABLE POTPOURRI

2 medium onions, thinly sliced
2 large cloves garlic, crushed
2 tablespoons olive oil
1 medium eggplant cut into
 ½-inch cubes
2 medium tomatoes, peeled
 and diced
1 medium green pepper,
 cut into strips

1 small yellow squash, cut into
 1½-inch strips
1 medium potato, diced
1 cup nonfat chicken broth
½ teaspoon salt
¼ teaspoon fresh ground black
 pepper

In Dutch oven sauté onions and garlic in hot oil until tender, about 5–7 minutes. Stir in all of the vegetables, broth, salt, and pepper; bring to a boil. Cover and simmer, stirring occasionally, 20–25 minutes or until liquid has been absorbed.
Serves 5
Exchanges= 1 starch, 1 vegetable

WHOLE WHEAT RAISIN BREAD

2–3 cups all-purpose white flour
½ cup sugar
3 teaspoons salt
1 teaspoon cinnamon
½ teaspoon nutmeg
2 pkg active dry yeast
2 cups milk

¾ cup water
¼ cup vegetable oil
4 cups whole-wheat flour
1 cup rolled oats
1 cup raisins
1 tablespoon butter, melted

In mixing large bowl combine 1½ cups all-purpose flour, ½ cup sugar, cinnamon, nutmeg, and yeast; mix well.

In medium pan, heat milk, water, and oil until very warm (120–130°F). Add warm liquid to flour mixture; blend with mixer at low speed just until moistened. Beat at medium speed.

By hand, stir in whole-wheat flour, rolled oats, raisins and an additional ¼ to ¾ cup all-purpose flour until dough pulls cleanly away from sides of bowl.

On floured surface, knead in remaining ¼ to ¾ cup all-purpose flour until dough is smooth and elastic, about 5 minutes. Place dough in large greased bowl; cover loosely with greased plastic wrap and cloth towel. Let rise in warm place (80–85°F.) until light and doubled in size, 20–30 minutes.

Grease two 9 x 5 loaf pans.

Punch down dough several times to remove air bubbles. Divide dough in half; shape into loaves. Place in greased pans; cover and let rise in warm place until light and doubled in size, 30–45 minutes.

Heat oven to 375°F. Uncover dough. Place pans in oven and bake 40–50 minutes or until deep golden brown and loaves sound hollow when lightly tapped. Immediately remove from pans and cool on racks for 1½ hours or until completely cooled. Brush tops of loaves with melted butter; sprinkle with sugar.

Makes 2 loaves. Serving size = 1 slice. Exchanges = 2 starch.

SCALLOPED CORN BAKE

¼ cup margarine or butter
½ cup finely chopped onion
½ green bell pepper, finely chopped
½ red bell pepper, finely chopped
1 (15 oz) can creamed corn
½ cup Italian seasoned dry
  bread crumbs
2 eggs, beaten

Heat oven to 375°F. Grease a one-quart baking dish.
In medium saucepan, melt margarine or butter over medium heat. Add onion and bell pepper; cook 3–4 minutes or until crisp-tender.

Stir in remaining ingredients. Pour into prepared baking dish.

Bake 375°F. for 35–40 minutes or until knife inserted in center comes out clean.

Serves 6 (½ cup servings). Exchanges = 1 starch, 1 vegetable, 2 fat

CRANBERRY BREAD

2 eggs
¼ cup water
12 slices dry bread, rolled into crumbs
⅔ cup dry powdered milk
1 teaspoon grated orange peel
1 teaspoon vanilla extract

¼ teaspoon baking soda
2 cups fresh or frozen
  cranberries
Artificial sweetener to
  equal 6 teaspoons sugar

Combine all ingredients except cranberries in blender; whip for 1 minute. Add this mixture to a large bowl containing the cranberries. Mix well.

Pour mixture into a 10-inch nonstick-surface baking pan. Bake at 350°F. for 35–40 minutes, until top is puffed and light brown. Remove from pan and cool on rack.
Cut loaf into 9 slices.
Exchanges = 1 starch

SLOPPY JOES

1 pound extra-lean ground beef
½ cup finely chopped onion
½ cup finely chopped green bell
  pepper
1 tablespoon brown sugar
1 teaspoon dry mustard
¼ teaspoon salt

½ cup ketchup
1 tablespoon cider vinegar
1 tablespoon Worcestershire
  sauce
1 (8 oz) can tomato sauce
6 sandwich buns

In large skillet, combine ground beef, onion, and green pepper; sauté over medium heat for 8–10 minutes or until beef is thoroughly cooked. Drain well.

Add remaining ingredients, except for buns; mix well. Cover and simmer 15–20 minutes, stirring frequently. Serve on buns.
Serves 6
Exchanges = 1½ starch, 1 vegetable, 2 medium-fat meat

SALMON CROQUETTES

1 (3 oz) can salmon, drained and flaked
1 teaspoon dehydrated onion flakes
4 tablespoons finely chopped celery
prepared mustard, enough to moisten

Preheat oven to 350°F.
    Mix all ingredients and make into patties.
    Place on foil; bake 20 minutes in 350°F. oven. Then broil until brown.
Serves 1
Exchanges = 2 very-lean meat

OVEN-FRIED CHICKEN

1½ cups very finely crushed cornflakes
1 teaspoon seasoned salt
½ teaspoon paprika
¼ teaspoon garlic powder
¼ teaspoon black pepper

¼ cup margarine or butter, melted
1 tablespoon water
1 egg
2 pounds frying chicken parts, skin removed

Heat oven to 400°F. In large bowl combine all dry ingredients. Add margarine; mix well. In another bowl beat egg and water.
    Dip chicken pieces in egg mixture; coat all sides with cornflake mixture. Place chicken in greased 13 x 9 baking dish.
    Bake at 400°F. for 55–60 minutes or until chicken is fork tender and juices run clear.
Serves 8 (with 4 oz meat per serving).
Exchanges = 4 lean meat, 1½ starch, ½ fat

ROASTED CHICKEN IN GARDEN VEGETABLES

¼ cup flour
¼ teaspoon fresh ground black
  pepper
¼ teaspoon salt
2 pounds frying chicken parts,
  skin removed
1 tablespoons olive oil
2 large garlic cloves, minced
1 large onion, sliced

2 medium tomatoes, chopped
  coarsely
1 red bell pepper, cut into
  slices
1 medium zucchini, sliced
1 medium yellow summer
  squash, sliced
1 tablespoon chopped fresh
  basil

In plastic bag, mix flour, salt, and pepper. Add chicken pieces to bag; shake to coat.

Heat oil in large skillet until hot. Add chicken; fry until brown on all sides.

Remove chicken from skillet. Add onion and garlic; cook until tender. Add tomatoes; return chicken to skillet. Cover and cook over medium-low heat for 30 minutes.

Add bell pepper, zucchini, yellow squash; cover and cook an additional 5–10 minutes or until chicken is fork-tender, juices run clear, and vegetables are crisp-tender.

Remove chicken from skillet; place on serving platter. Add basil to skillet; mix well. Serve vegetables over chicken.

Serves 8 (4 oz meat per serving)
Exchanges = 1 starch, 2 vegetable, 4 very-lean meat, 1 fat

APPLESAUCE MEATLOAF

2 pounds ground round
1 cup unsweetened applesauce
1 onion, finely chopped
1 green bell pepper, fined chopped
6 slices whole-grain bread, finely crumbled

1 egg
2 teaspoons salt
pepper to taste
½ cup tomato sauce

Preheat oven to 350°F.

Combine all ingredients except tomato sauce. With hand,

knead mixture until well blended. Pack into loaf pan. Pour tomato sauce over top. Bake for 2 hours.

Turn out of pan and slice in to 8 sections.

Serves 8. Exchanges = 4 very-lean meat, 1 starch, ½ fruit

BROWN GRAHAM BREAD

2 cups whole-wheat flour
1 cup all-purpose white flour
½ cup corn meal
¼ cup sugar
2 teaspoons baking soda

1 teaspoon baking powder
1 teaspoon salt
½ cup molasses
2 cups sour milk
1 cup raisins

Mix all dry ingredients in large bowl. Blend in molasses and sour milk. Fold in raisins.

Pour batter into 2 small well-greased loaf pans.

Bake at 350°F. for 35-40 minutes.

One loaf makes 15 slices.

Serving = 1 slice. Exchanges = 1 bread/starch

ROASTED GARLIC CHICKEN

2 pounds frying chicken pieces,
  skin removed
3 tablespoons margarine or butter,
  melted
1 tablespoon dried parsley flakes

2 tablespoons soy sauce
1 teaspoon corn starch
¼ teaspoon powdered ginger
4–6 large cloves garlic, minced

Preheat oven to 350°F. Put chicken pieces in greased 12 x 8 inch baking dish.

Combine remaining ingredients in small bowl. Brush chicken with soy sauce mixture.

Bake at 350°F. for 45–55 minutes or until chicken is fork-tender and juice runs clear. Baste with drippings halfway through baking.

Serves 8 (4 oz meat per serving). Exchanges= 4 very-lean meat, ½ fat

OUR FAVORITE
BRAN MUFFINS

2 cups whole bran cereal
2½ cups buttermilk
½ cup vegetable oil
2 eggs
2½ cups all-purpose white flour

1½ cups sugar
1¼ teaspoons baking soda
1 teaspoon baking powder
½ teaspoon salt
¾ cups raisins

Preheat oven to 400°F.

Combine thoroughly cereal and buttermilk in large bowl. Let stand 5 minutes until cereal is softened. Add oil and eggs; blend well.

Grease muffin cups; fill cups ¾ full.

Bake at 400°F. for 18–20 minutes or until toothpick inserted in center comes out clean. Immediately remove from pan.

(Note: Batter can be stored in refrigerator for up to 2 weeks.)
Makes 30 muffins. Serving = 1 muffin
Exchanges = 1 starch, ½ fruit, ½ fat

GOOD OLD YANKEE
POT ROAST

3 pounds chuck roast of beef
1 large onion, sliced
   lemon pepper
1 package brown gravy mix

3 tablespoons red wine
10 medium potatoes
10 medium carrots, pared and
   cut in chunks

Preheat oven to 350°F.

Arrange beef in a large casserole. Place onion on beef. Sprinkle with lemon pepper and gravy mix. Pour wine over top.

Cover and roast in 350-degree oven.

Add carrots and potatoes the last 45–60 minutes of cooking (total cooking time: 2½–3 hours).
Serves 8 (4 oz meat per serving).
Exchanges = 4 medium fat meat, 1 starch (1 potato), 1 vegetable
(½ cup carrots)

BREAKFAST COBBLER

1 egg
½ cup skim milk
1 diced apple
1 slice bread, crumbled
½ teaspoon vanilla

⅛ teaspoon cinnamon
⅛ teaspoon butter
¼ teaspoon almond flavoring
artificial sweetener to taste

Beat egg.
  Add skim milk, crumbled bread, diced apple, and flavoring.
  Pour into small baking dish.
  Bake 20 minutes at 350°F.
  Sprinkle with sweetener on top.
Serves 1
Exchanges = 1 meat, 1 bread/starch, 1 fruit, ½ milk, 1 fat

SHRIMP SALAD SANDWICHES

8 ounces cooked shrimp, chopped
¾ cup finely chopped celery
⅔ cup non-fat mayonnaise
1 tablespoon minced onion
½ teaspoon crushed, dried tarragon
4 hot dog rolls
lettuce or spinach leaves

In medium bowl, combine first five ingredients; mix well.
Refrigerate for at least an hour. Place lettuce or spinach
leaves into each roll. Spoon ½ cup mixture into each roll.
Serves 4
Exchanges= 2 very-lean meat, 1½ starch, ½ fat

GERMAN POTATO SALAD

2 pounds small new red potatoes
4 slices bacon, cooked crisp
2 tablespoons reserved bacon fat drippings
½ cup finely chopped onion
¼ cup sugar

2 tablespoons flour
½ teaspoon salt
pepper to taste
1 cup water
⅓ cup cider vinegar

Cook potatoes in medium saucepan until tender. Drain, cool, and slice.

In reserved bacon drippings sauté onion until crisp-tender.

Add sugar, flour, salt, and pepper to sautéed onions; blend well. Gradually add water and vinegar. Cook over medium high heat until bubbly and thickened, stirring constantly.

Stir in potatoes; cook until thoroughly heated. Crumble bacon; sprinkle on top.

Serves 8 (½-cup servings).

Exchanges = 1½ starch, 1 fat

APPLE SALAD

3 medium Red Delicious apples, unpeeled and cut into chunks
½ cup crushed pineapple, drained (reserve juice)
¼ cup celery, diced
2 tablespoons raisins

3 tablespoons plain nonfat yogurt
2 tablespoons mayonnaise
1 tablespoon pineapple juice
1 tablespoon lemon juice
½ teaspoon cinnamon

Combine apples, pineapple, celery, and raisins.

Mix remaining ingredients. Fold apple mixture into yogurt mixture.

Serves 10.

Exchanges = 1 fruit, ½ fat

TUNA MELT

3 ounces water-packed tuna
1 teaspoon lemon juice
finely chopped celery and onion to taste

2 slices pineapple
1 ounce any low-fat cheese
1 English muffin, toasted

Mash tuna and moisten with lemon juice. Add onion and celery.

Place one pineapple ring on each muffin half.

Cover with cheese and broil.

Serves 2.

Exchanges = 2 meat, 1 starch, 1 fruit, 1 fat

EGGS, SOUTHWESTERN STYLE

¾ pound spicy low-fat pork sausage, bulk style
½ cup finely chopped onion
½ cup finely chopped red and green bell pepper
4 cups refrigerated or frozen hash-brown potatoes, thawed
6 oz (1½ cups) low-fat shredded cheddar cheese
4 eggs
¾ cup skim milk
1 cup chunky salsa—you pick the spiciness

Preheat oven to 350°F. Grease an 8-inch square baking dish. In medium skillet sauté sausage, onion, and bell pepper until browned. Drain.

Arrange potatoes in bottom of greased baking dish. Top with half of the cheese, all of the sausage mixture, and the remaining cheese.

Beat eggs in small bowl. Beat in milk. Pour egg mixture over sausage mixture. Cover with foil.

Bake at 350°F. for 1 hour. Uncover and bake an additional 10–15 minutes. Let stand 5 minutes before serving. Serve with salsa.

Serves 6.

Exchanges= 1½ starch, 2½ medium-fat meat, 1 fat

ORANGE BAKED CHICKEN

6 boneless, skinless chicken breast halves
¼ cup orange juice
1 teaspoon grated orange peel
2 tablespoons soy sauce
½ teaspoon ground cinnamon, ginger, or curry powder
pepper to taste

Preheat oven to 350°F.

Place chicken breasts in 13 x 9 x 2-inch baking dish. Combine all other ingredients and pour over chicken.

Cover and refrigerate about 2 hours.

Bake at 350°F. for 45–60 minutes.

Serves 6.

Exchanges = 4 very-lean meat

PORK TENDERLOIN WITH HONEY MUSTARD SAUCE

1 tablespoon honey
1 tablespoon Dijon mustard
2 teaspoons olive oil

2 large garlic cloves, minced
½ teaspoon dried oregano leaves
1 (¾ pound) pork tenderloin

Preheat oven to 425°F. Line baking dish large enough to hold tenderloin with foil.

In small bowl, combine all other ingredients. Brush tenderloin with mustard/honey mixture; place on foil lined baking dish.

Bake at 425°F. for 25–30 minutes or until pork is no longer pink in center. Let stand for 5 minutes. Slice into 4 servings

Serves 4.

Exchanges = ½ starch, 2 lean meat

HERB AND MUSHROOM RICE

1 (10½ oz) can nonfat beef or chicken broth
1 (4 oz) can sliced mushrooms, drained, reserving liquid
2 medium onions, chopped
½ cup wild rice
1 cup long grain rice
2 tablespoons parsley

Add water to broth to make 2 cups. Boil broth, mushroom liquid, and onions in saucepan.

Add wild rice, reduce heat; simmer 20 minutes.

Add regular rice and mushrooms. Boil again; simmer 20 minutes until tender.

Garnish with parsley.
Serves 10 (½ cup each).
Exchanges = 1 starch, 1 vegetable

BEST POTATO SOUP EVER

4 large baking potatoes
4 slices bacon, fried crisp, save drippings
6 cups low fat milk
½ cup flour
4 green onions, sliced
1¼ cups shredded sharp low-fat Cheddar cheese
¾ teaspoon salt
pepper to taste
1 cup nonfat sour cream

Bake potatoes in oven or microwave. Cool slightly.

In large saucepan, mix flour in bacon drippings; add milk and blend well. Cook over medium heat until bubbly and thickened, stirring constantly.

Scoop out potato from skins (can discard or save skins for another use); put in medium bowl and mash potatoes well. Add potatoes, bacon, onions, cheese, salt, and pepper. Cook until cheese is melted. Add sour cream; cook and stir until soup is thoroughly heated.
Serves 7 (1½ cups)
Exchanges = 2½ starch, 1½ medium-fat meat, 1 fat

MID-EASTERN SANDWICHES

1 (15 oz) can garbanzo beans,
  rinsed, drained
¼ cup sesame seed
⅛ teaspoon cayenne pepper
2 tablespoons lemon juice

2 tablespoons water
3 large cloves garlic, minced
8 slices rye bread
1 large tomato, sliced
1 cup alfalfa sprouts

In food processor, combine beans, sesame seed, cayenne pepper, lemon juice, water, and garlic; process until smooth. Cover and refrigerate at least an hour to marry flavors.

Generously spread 4 slices with bean mixture. Top with slice of tomato, sprouts, and other bread slices.
Serves 4.
Exchanges = 3 starch, ½ very-lean meat, 1 fat

BEEF–CABBAGE CASSEROLE

1 pound lean ground beef
1 onion, finely chopped
4 ounces tomato sauce
4–7 ounces tomato juice

⅛ teaspoon cinnamon
⅛ teaspoon ground cloves
4 cups shredded cabbage

Brown meat and drain off all fat. Mix onion, tomato sauce and juice, cinnamon, and cloves; add to beef.

Put 2 cups of shredded cabbage in bottom of 2-quart baking dish.

Top with half of the meat mixture. Add last of cabbage and last of meat in the next 2 layers.

Cover and bake at 350°F. for 45 minutes.
Serves 4.
Exchanges = 4 lean meat, 2 vegetable, ½ fat

WAKE-UP SHAKE

1 cup cranberry juice
2 ripe bananas, sliced
2 cartons (8 oz each) nonfat raspberry yogurt
artificial sweetener to equal 1 tablespoon sugar

In blender, combine all ingredients; cover and blend at medium speed until smooth. Serve immediately.
Serves 4. Exchanges = 2 fruit, ½ skim milk

EASY VEGETABLE SOUP

1½ pounds lean ground beef
½ cup chopped onions
½ cup diced potatoes
½ cup sliced carrots
½ cup chopped celery
½ cup shredded cabbage
1 cup canned chopped tomatoes

3 cups water
⅛ cup rice
1 bay leaf
¼ teaspoon thyme
½ teaspoon dried basil
2 teaspoons salt
pepper to taste

Cook ground beef and onions in skillet until meat is brown; drain meat and blot with paper towels to remove rest of grease.

Combine meat and remaining ingredients in large pot. Simmer until vegetables are tender.
Serves 6. Exchanges= 2 meat, 1 starch, 2 vegetable, 1 fat

VEGGIE STIR-FRY

1 cup broccoli, sliced
1 cup onions, in small wedges
½ pound fresh mushrooms, sliced

1 red bell pepper, in strips
1 pkg seasoned chicken broth

Mix a little water with dry chicken broth in large skillet. Heat skillet to high; add vegetables and stir-fry till tender.
Serves 6. Exchanges = 2 vegetable

Discipline

The second emphasis in this program is on discipline. So often the word discipline connotes a negative response in us, and we forget that it is a positive action necessary for Christian growth. Hebrews tells us that discipline is painful rather than pleasant (for the moment), but it promises to produce the fruit of righteousness to those of us who will be trained by it (Heb. 12:11).

Take a new look at the word discipline and let God change your opinion about it. It will set you free.

Since God desires us to lead well-ordered and disciplined lives, the disciplines of the 3D program will serve as tools to help you develop new habit patterns in prayer, Bible study, eating, work, use of time, and caring for others. Each discipline is an important part of 3D's goal to help you become the person God wants you to be.

Prayer

Daily prayer will help you develop a closer relationship with God. Praying consistently at a regular time each day will help reinforce your prayer discipline. It only takes a minute or two to bring ten names to the Lord. He knows their specific needs, but praying for others deeply blesses us in the process. If you are in a group, pray for the other members as well as the leaders every day for twelve weeks. You will be amazed at how exciting it is to be a small part of what God does for the members of the group. If you are doing 3D alone, pray for five people you know (other than family). Make a commitment to God to faithfully pray for them each day.

"My Prayer List"
1.
2.
3.
4.
5.

This is also a good time to pray for your family, your church, the country, your personal needs, and other concerns which the Lord may bring to mind. Pray expectantly—God's answers are exciting!

ATTENDANCE AT GROUP MEETINGS

Faithful weekly attendance is an important element of your commitment to the program. Since the 3D group is a safe place in which inner conflicts can be faced, exposed, fought, and healed, the support of the group is vital.

If you are doing this program on your own, it would be our recommendation that you decide before starting the twelve weeks, the day and time of the week you are going to weigh yourself. Also, remember to set a daily specific time for your prayer, daily devotional reading, and Bible study. This will require discipline on your part since you do not have the support of a group around you.

Daily Devotional Readings and Bible Study

Daily devotional readings and Bible study questions are a very important part of the 3D program. Whenever we deny ourselves, whether it is by being on a diet or getting up in the morning earlier than usual, we find ourselves more rebellious than we even imagined. Being "fed" spiritually by daily devotions, Bible reading, and Bible study is a vital part of what God wants to do for you during these next twelve weeks. Don't miss this part of the program. Your journal is included in this packet.

The Food Sheet

Each day record all that you eat on your food sheet. We would encourage you to record each meal as you eat rather than once a day. The food sheet should be turned into the 3D leaders at your group meeting time.

There is a possibility that you have never been this honest about your eating habits. We pray that this record will show you the trouble spots in your day and where you need to change. Then you can ask Jesus to help you.

This food sheet can be a valuable tool even if you are not interested in losing weight. It helps you see weak areas in your eating patterns and where you are not receiving good nutrition. It is also an excellent tool for anyone suffering from eating disorders.

Menu Planning

Menu planning is an area where discipline is frequently lacking. Too often a family eats meals that reflect the mood of the cook. Do not allow poor preparation or planning to be an excuse for disobedience. You will be blessed by a carefully planned menu.

God is concerned about your stewardship in the use of money and time. By making out a menu and shopping list ahead of time, you can check advertisements and clip coupons. Include specials in the menus to help keep within your food budget.

BIBLE MEMORIZATION

The Psalmist said, "I have laid up thy word in my heart, that I might not sin against thee" (Psalm 119:11).

The Word of God will strengthen, encourage, and protect you as you face the problems and temptations of daily living. To help you put God's Word in your heart, Bible memorization is part of 3D. Each week memorize the verse corresponding to the lesson of the week, and then commit it to your heart so that you may practice it daily. The verse is found at the beginning of each week in your devotional workbook.

CARING FOR ANOTHER

Too often we become concerned with our own problems, which grow out of proportion and are overwhelming. Serving and caring for others helps us keep our problems in perspective. One telephone call or a visit with someone each week is a way to begin this.

Be open to the prompting of the Holy Spirit in making telephone calls. He can show you whom to call and when to make the call. We encourage people in 3D to make one "caring" call each week, or a visit. Be sensitive to the time of day you make your call, and the length of each conversation. *Don't talk too long*!

Try to serve others in your contacts with those in your group and don't hesitate to share your own needs in these conversations.

If you are doing 3D on your own, ask the Lord to lead you in a caring deed every week for someone else. It can be a phone call, or a letter to someone, or a visit to a shut-in.

Exercise

3D is concerned about the whole area of exercise—not only for weight loss but for overall good health purposes. However, we also feel exercise can be overdone and needs to be carefully considered for each individual.

Lasting Benefits of Physical Activity

Edward J. Haver, MA, FAACVPR
Director of the Cardiac Rehabilitation Program,
Charleston Area Medical Center,
Charleston, West Virginia.
Exercise Consultant to 3D

What kind of visual picture do you get when you hear the word "exercise"? Do you see people sweating, panting and pushing until they are close to collapse? Or, do you picture a Marine drill sergeant barking out, "one, two, three, four . . ." as you try to keep up with calisthenics that must have come from a book of medieval tortures? As you read this, I'd like to have you clear your head of any negative thoughts that you might have. Be sure to hang on to any positive ones, and for the next few minutes let me convince you that exercise is the greatest thing since sliced bread.

The human body was made to be active. When God designed our bodies, He planned that they would function at their peak efficiency in an environment of movement. As you study the life of Jesus, you find no examples of structured exercise periods, yet how many of us could walk from Galilee to Jerusalem (75 miles one way), as He often did? For that matter, how many of us could walk from Jerusalem up the hill to the Garden of Gethsemane?

Even as recently as 60 years ago, the vast majority of Americans (and most of the world even today) spent most of their day in physical labor. There was no need for them to ride the stationary bike for 30 minutes when they got home. With our modern technology, we have numerous laborsaving devices that, while saving us time, have ruined our health. Primary among the negative end result is coronary heart disease, which kills more women and men than all other causes of death combined. In the last 60 years there has also been a significant increase in diabetes, stroke, hypertension, obesity, depression, anxiety, osteoporosis and other diseases related to a sedentary lifestyle. Our bodies are tremendous gifts designed and given to us by God, and it is our responsibility to take care of them. Physical activity is an integral part of the 3D program not only because it has been shown to help in weight loss, but primarily because it helps our bodies function as God intended.

The Surgeon General issued a report on Physical Activity and Health in 1996 that concluded that regular exercise significantly reduces the risk of developing or

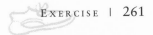

dying from some of the leading causes of death in the U.S., including:

- heart disease
- stroke
- diabetes
- high blood pressure
- colon cancer

In addition, regular physical activity has been shown to:

- help build and maintain healthy bones and prevent osteoporosis
- reduce feelings of depression and anxiety
- increase resistance to disease and fatigue
- help cope with stress
- help control weight
- improve quality of sleep
- increase muscle tone
- improve posture
- increase resistance to injury

I am convinced that the Lord wants His people to have bodies that function as He designed them, not plagued by problems brought about by our own neglect. Our desire to please the One who made us and bought us, and to "honor God with your bodies" (1 Corinthians 6:20), should be reason enough for us to get moving!

Physical Activity and Weight Loss

The good news is that the Surgeon General's report also called physical activity the "key component of any weight loss effort and important for controlling weight." Research is showing over and over again what any dieter will tell you—it is very difficult to diet your way permanently to a healthy weight. Long-term success is based on adopting a lifestyle that incorporates regular physical activity.

Physical activity does much more than just burn calories—although there is nothing wrong with that! It also changes how your body burns calories all through the day and night, improves the ratio of lean body weight to fat weight, often decreases your appetite, helps you lose weight in the most important places, and complements the benefits of a good food plan.

To achieve permanent weight loss it helps to understand the role of your resting metabolic rate or RMR. Your RMR is that rate at which your body burns calories while you are at rest, keeping all of your body functions going. As you go on a "diet" and limit your caloric intake, your body often interprets this reduction as starvation, and your RMR will decrease as your body works to preserve itself. In extreme cases, even your hair and fingernails will stop growing as your body works to conserve energy. Therefore, the low-calorie diet that has you losing pounds at the beginning, a few weeks later might simply maintain your weight. I can't think of anything that is more discouraging than to work hard counting calories only to have your body work just as hard to decrease how many it burns. In addition, up to 25 percent of what you lose will not be fat but lean body weight, primarily muscle, which is the very thing that keeps your RMR going. Worse yet, when you go back to "regular" eating your RMR will still be in its survival mode and it will continue to burn calories more slowly to prepare for the next famine (diet) by putting away fat. That is why someone can gain weight back so quickly after months of working to get rid of it. Is there any doubt as to why the obesity rates have doubled in the U.S. over the past 10 years in the midst of people spending billions on the latest diet books? However, by adding regular physical activity to your weight loss plan, many of these problems can be counteracted. You can increase your muscle mass and lose primarily fat, keep your RMR from dropping, burn excess calories for hours following physical activity, and be successful in achieving long-term weight loss.

Increasing Your Physical Activity

The goal of a good physical activity plan is to help you improve your overall health. You might have noticed that I have tried to avoid using the "E" word, exercise, to describe what is important. After several decades of trying to get people to exercise, and having little success, it has been realized that the more realistic goal is to get people to move. If you haven't been active recently it is important that you begin slowly, and gradually build up. If you have chronic health problems, such as heart disease, diabetes, or obesity, you should first consult with your physician. This might sound like the typical line—and it is, but it's important to let your doctor know what you're doing to minimize the risks and maximize the benefits.

Your long-term goal should be to accumulate 30 minutes or more of moderate physical activity on most days of the week—*for the rest of your life!* It's important to not get overwhelmed with the "journey," but just to begin with the first step—and take it today! The main reason given by most people for why they can't "exercise" is that they just don't have the time. New research has shown the value of *accumulated* activity, meaning ten minutes here, five minutes there, all counts! And the emphasis is on physical *activity*, which includes taking the stairs, mowing the lawn, mopping the floor, or walking across the parking lot. As Americans we have been trained to think in terms of conserving our energy and saving steps, and you need to learn to begin to think in just the opposite way— how much energy can you spend during the day? Park farther away, take the stairs instead of the elevator, take a short walk during a coffee break—keep looking for ways to incorporate more movement into what you're already doing.

If you have a sedentary job you might still find it difficult to accumulate 30 minutes (or up to 60 minutes for weight loss) of activity throughout the day. Most of us need to add some kind of structured activity if we are going to reach these goals. This might be walking, swimming, an aerobics class, bicycling, or using a variety of exercise equipment at home or at a health club. Many people find it easier to start at home— there are many good Christian exercise videos that you can do in the privacy of your own home, wearing what you want and not worrying about anyone else. On the following pages you will find a set of general toning exercises that you can begin to do to help tone the muscles in your arms, waist, legs, hips, and middle. Remember to start slowly with these and gradually increase to the numbers mentioned with the diagrams. You could also begin by simply walking in the house— many of the patients I work with have figured out walking routes going throughout their homes, the only drawback is that you might wear out the carpet! This kind of activity can seem very "artificial" or "unnatural," but you have to remember that the unnatural activity is sitting all day! The goal is to replace what has been removed from our lives; a combination of an increasingly active lifestyle *and* some regular structured activities is usually the answer.

One question people often ask is how "hard" they have to work to benefit from exercise. In our society we tend to want to "give it all we've got"—and get it over with as quickly as possible! Instead, we should think in terms of activities that can be sustained fairly comfortably for a long period of time—forget the "no pain, no gain" motto! Generally, after an initial warm-up period, you shouldn't be out of breath; if you're finding yourself constantly breathing hard, try an easier pace. If you are walking or exercising with someone else, you should be able to talk as you move along. On the other hand, if you are moving so slowly that you are questioning if it is helpful, try picking up the pace and use the "talk test" as a gauge. You should finish a session of walking or other activity feeling refreshed, not exhausted—even if your muscles are letting you know that they have been working for you!

Important Parts of an Activity Program

Whatever activity you are going to do, it is important to follow a few guidelines. Just as you warm up your car for a few minutes on a cold day, you need to warm up your body. You are asking it to make numerous changes—heart rate, blood pressure, breathing rate, blood flow, muscle activity—every time you step up the pace. At the least you need to begin slowly and take a minute or two to get up to your cruising speed. The ideal is to warm up a little and then stretch for a couple of minutes to get all of your muscles and joints and their connections ready to safely move. Stretching is a great activity whether or not it is followed by another activity, but it is especially important at the beginning of an exercise session. In this book you will find drawings of several basic stretching exercises that are especially helpful for increasing your flexibility. Remember to hold each stretch for a count of at least five and keep breathing while you are stretching! These basic eight will take approximately four minutes to complete and should become a part of your daily routine. Doing these stretches regularly will decrease your chance of injury as you increase your level of activity.

At the other end of your activity, just like a horse after a horse race, you need to cool down after you're finished. This can be as simple as slowing down and not stopping suddenly. When you are working your body, there are many, many positive changes occurring to meet the demands you are placing on it. The blood is pumping faster through your body to feed the muscles that are requiring oxygen that is coming from your increased breathing. Much of this blood supply is probably going to the muscles in your legs since they are doing much of the work. The blood has to get back to your heart and it does this by traveling up the veins in your legs. The veins depend on the muscles around them contracting to squeeze the blood against gravity. If you suddenly stop, these muscle pumps stop and the blood tends to pool in your legs, causing your blood pressure to drop rapidly. This puts more demand on your heart to try to maintain the blood pressure. If you have ever felt dizzy after you after exercised hard it was probably due to stopping too quickly. You need to keep moving and gradually slow down. This is a great time to do the stretching exercises, as your muscles, tendons and ligaments are warmed up and ready to stretch. Remember to warm up and cool down if you are doing an activity that will last more than 20 minutes. For activities of a short duration, you might just warm up and cool down!

Overcoming Barriers to Keeping Moving

There are many daily challenges that we all face that will tend to sidetrack the best of intentions. As you make physical activity part of your lifestyle, you will need to be creative. Some of the ideas that have helped other people overcome these barriers include:

- **Plan ahead.** If you are going to exercise in the morning (a good time for consistency), you need to get everything laid out the night before and be ready to go without too much thought. The idea is to get up and out the door before your brain wakes up! No matter when you plan an exercise session, you need to fill it in on your schedule and keep the appointment.
- **Exercise with a friend.** This is great for your friend as well as you! The Bible says that two are better than one, and that is definitely true of exercise. The accountability of another person or group can really make a difference. This is a great time for sharing and encouraging each other—remember that talking is allowed!
- **Find an activity that is "fun."** You should enjoy what you are doing, even if the enjoyment comes from having done it! It is important that this not be

a time of torture. If it is, then find something else you can do.

- **Get into a routine.** The regularity of exercising at the same time on the same days of the week leads to the development of a habit that is harder to break. Include as much variety as you like, but make it as consistent as possible until it becomes an integral part of your life.

- **Look for opportunities to be active during the day.** Take the stairs, park further away (and save time not circling the parking lot), do calisthenics or stretches (some of these are diagramed on the following pages) while watching your favorite show, or pull out that old exercise equipment for the days when you can't get out.

- **Be flexible.** If you find your exercise becomes sporadic, stop and analyze the reasons why. Getting up at 6 AM might have been fine during the summer—but bring on the dark and cold of winter and motivation can wear thin. Can you plug in some activity at lunchtime, or possibly in the afternoon? Don't let minor problems sidetrack your efforts—look at them as opportunities to be creative.

- **Buy a pedometer.** One of the best ways to keep track of what you are doing is a simple little gadget called a pedometer. These have been around for years but are now making a comeback as a way to keep track of steps taken during the day. This little device has helped motivate many people to get in their daily steps (with a stated goal of 10,000).

- **Involve your family.** There is nothing better than being active with your spouse or kids. My wife has been my jogging partner for 28 years and we keep each other going (plus have some good discussions while we run), and our daughters have both become exercisers as well.

- **Memorize Bible verses.** Especially meditate on ones that relate to taking care of your body (1 Corinthians 9:24–26), using what God has given you wisely (Matthew 25:20 and Luke 19:16), correct motives (1 Corinthians 4:5), or any other verses that give you strength and encouragement. You can also post verses around the house to boost your motivation.
- **Pray.** If God wants you to do this, He is ready to give you the discipline and desire to make it happen, and He can even make it fun!

STRETCHING EXERCISES

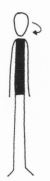

1. *Neck Stretch*: Look over left shoulder, back to middle, look over right shoulder. Hold at each position, repeat 5 times.

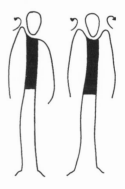

2. *Shoulder Rolls*: Lift and rotate right shoulder back, lift and rotate left shoulder back, lift and rotate both shoulders back together. Repeat for a total of 4 times.

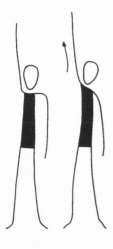

3. *Reach to Heaven*: Raise right arm over head, left arm down at your side, stretch and extend the right arm. Then switch and repeat the stretch and extend movement with the left arm up and right arm down. Repeat for a total of 8.

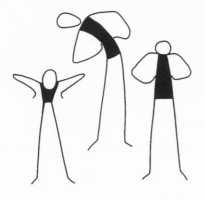

4. *Waist Rolls*: Place hands on hips, legs shoulder width apart. Bend forward at the waist, rotate body right, back, left and forward. Repeat. Then reverse and rotate body left, back, right and forward. Repeat.

5. *Lean Stretch*: Stand up straight, with feet shoulder width apart, and extend arms shoulder height with palms facing out toward the walls. Alternate pushing toward the wall with palms by leaning first right, then left. Alternate this movement for a total of 8.

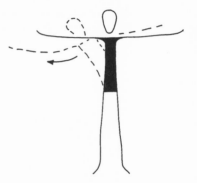

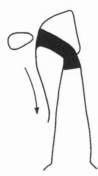

6. *Slide Stretch*: Keep feet shoulder width apart, arms down at sides, bend to the right and slide arm down right leg, while left arm slides up. Repeat to the left. Do this exercise alternating sides for a total of 8. Remember to keep your stomach muscles pulled in tightly.

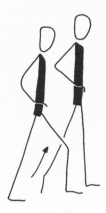

7. *Heel Stretch*: Stand with the left leg forward, knee bent, and right leg stretched behind as far back as needed to feel a stretch in the calf. The further behind the body you place the right leg, the greater the stretch. Then, raise and lower the right heel, stretching the calf muscle as you come down. Do 8 of these. Switch legs repeating the exercise with right leg forward, knee bent, and left leg behind for a total of 8.

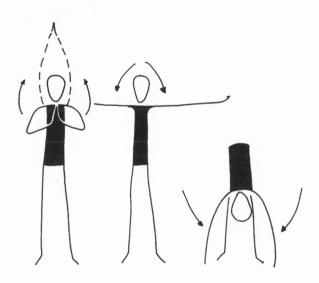

8. *Wake Up Praise*: Place palms together, lift arms up over head then separate and lower to sides as you bend over and sweep the floor. Repeat for a total of 4.

General Toning Exercises

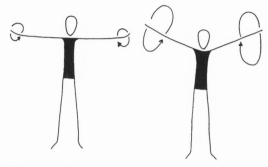

Arms

1. *Small and Large Arm Circles*: Stand with feet shoulder width apart, extend arms shoulder height and make 8 small circles forward and 8 small circles backwards and repeat. Follow this by making 4 large circles forward and 4 large circles backwards and repeat.

2. *Scissors*: Starting in a bent-over position, count to 8 while making a scissoring motion with arms, moving your body into a standing position with arms then up and over your head, then back down again to a count of 8 and repeat.

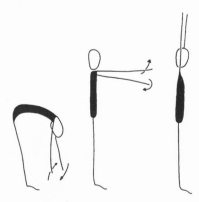

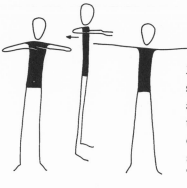

3. *Wing Stretches*: stand up straight and begin by bending arms so that fingers just touch at chest level. Stretch elbows back and then extend straightened arms back. There are 2 movements to each wing stretch and we do 16.

WAIST

1. *Wrap Arounds*: Feet shoulder width apart, extend arms and twist upper body to the right, wrapping the left arm around your waist. Twist left and wrap right arm around waist. Continue to alternate sides and do 16.

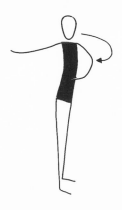

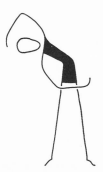

2. *Waist Reaches*: Pull stomach muscles tight, feet shoulder width apart and stretch left arm over head to the right and curve the right arm to the left in front. Reach and stretch for 8 times. Then repeat to the left 8 times.

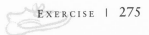

3. *Elbow Pulls*: Clasp hands
behind head and bend at the waist
to the right stretching to the count
8 times. Repeat on the left side.

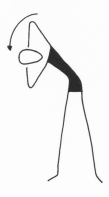

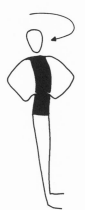

4. *Twists*: Place hands on hips
and twist upper body twice to the
right and then twist twice to the
left. There are 2 movements to
each "twist". Do a total of 16.

5. *Wood Chops*: Clasp hands
together over head, feet shoulder
width apart. Swing arms down
through legs, bending knees and
stretch arms through legs. Then,
swing arms back up over head.
Do a total of 8.

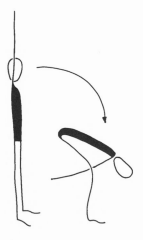

WAIST EXERCISES ON THE FLOOR:

1. *Waist and Inner Thigh Stretch*: Sit up straight on the floor, stomach pulled in, legs stretched open as wide as feels comfortable. Stretch left arm over head to the right and curve right arm to the left in front of you. Gently stretch 8 times. Then switch sides and repeat for a total of 8. (Shake out your legs.)

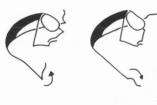

2. *Chest-to-Knee Stretch and Walk*: Legs stretched open wide, stretch down over right leg, hands on either side of leg. Do 8 stretches. Then "walk" your body using your hands, making 8 "steps" over to the left leg. Stretch eight times over the left leg. "Walk" back to the right leg and repeat. (Shake out your legs.)

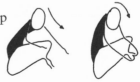

3. *Point and Flex*: With toes pointed, support the weight of your upper body on your hands. Lean body forward and stretch 8 times. Then flex feet and stretch forward 8 times. (Shake out your legs.)

4. *Inner Thigh Stretch*: Sit up straight, stomach pulled in, and bring the soles of your feet together in front of you, pulling feet as close to your body as is comfortable.

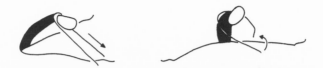

Then lean body forward for the stretch. For a gentler stretch, grab toes and lean body forward to each count. Or, for a deeper stretch, alternate arms extended in front of you and push palms forward. Do 16. (Shake out your legs.)

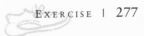

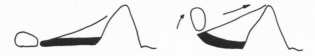

1. *Contractions*: Lie on back, knees slightly bent. Place hands on legs and lift shoulders off floor, pressing your back into the floor and contracting stomach muscles. Lie back and repeat. Do 8.

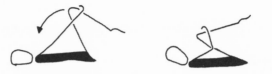

2. *Knee Hug*: Hug knees tightly to chest for 6 counts, then hold knees in a relaxed position of 6 counts and repeat.

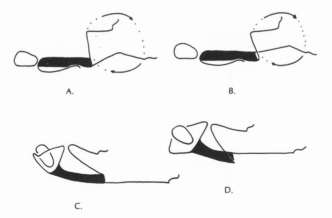

A.

B.

C.

D.

3. *Bicycle*: Lie on back with hands behind head, and bicycle legs for a total of 32 times. Try to keep legs as close to the floor as possible to better work the stomach muscles. If you have a bad back or haven't done any stomach exercises in a while, place your hands under the small of your back for support (A&B). For a more strenuous work out, alternate elbows to your knees (as in C&D).

4. *Stomach Stretch*: Lie on
back, with bent knees to
the left and arms to the

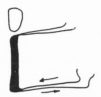

right over head, count to 8 and stretch and
release stomach muscles. Then switch sides, knees right
and arms left and repeat for 8 counts.

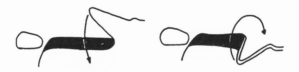

5. *Seat Walk*: Sitting up straight,
arms shoulder height in front of
you, "walk" your seat forward 8
counts and back 8 counts and
repeat 3 more times.

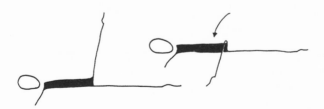

6. *Hip Rolls*: Lie on floor, arms spread shoulder height for
support, and bring knees to chest. Roll knees to the right,
come center, and roll left. Repeat for a total of 4 sets.

7. *Leg Crosses*: Lie on back with arms spread shoulder
height for support. Raise right leg waist level and cross leg
left over body, back up, and lower leg. Repeat with left leg
and continue for a total of 8.

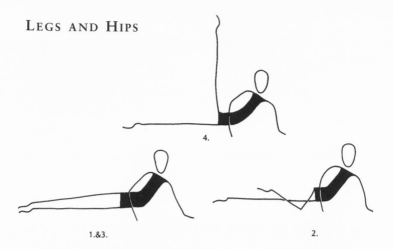

4.

1.&3.

2.

1. *Knee In-Leg Lifts*: Lie on left side, up on left elbow palms on the floor. Place both legs straight out with stomach pulled in and seat tucked under. Bend right knee into body, extend right leg, lift right leg straight up and lower. These 4 movements are one set. Do 8 sets. Roll over and repeat exercise working the left leg.

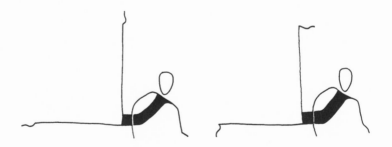

2. *Leg Lifts*: Lie on left side, up on elbow, palms on the floor, with both legs straight out, point toes and raise and lower right leg 8 times. Then flex the foot and raise and lower right leg 8 times. Roll over and repeat exercise working the left leg.

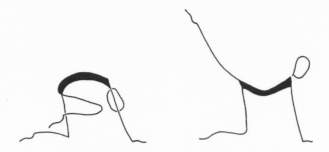

3. *Knee to Nose:* On hands and knees, bring right knee into chest, pulling head down. Then release leg back out and arch back while lifting head. Repeat for a total of 8 times. Then work the left leg 8 times.

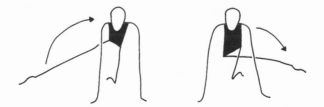

4. *Prayer Stretch:* Sit back on heels with arms stretched out in front. Next, lean forward and stretch up, supporting yourself on arms while letting the hips fall forward. Do this exercise 4 times.

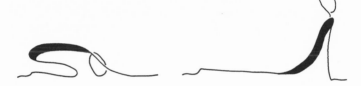

5. *Leg Swings:* On hands and knees, begin with the right leg out at almost a right angle to your body. Swing right leg to the left across the left leg and repeat. Do 8 of these and switch to work the left for a total of 8.

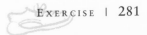

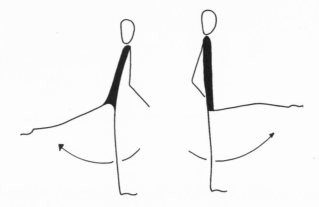

6. *Standing Leg Lifts*: Grab a chair, wall or pole, etc., for support, stand up straight, stomach pulled in with the right side of the body facing the chair. Swing the right leg forward and back for 8 counts. Then, turn around so that the left side of the body faces the chair, and repeat 8 counts with the left leg.

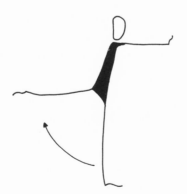

7. Next, face the chair and lift the right leg behind you for 8 counts and then work the left leg for 8 counts.

A Final Word about Discipline

As you have probably observed upon reading the material so far, 3D is a program with various phases which provide sound balance. You have just finished reading about one—exercise! Ed Haver's encouragement to exercise has no doubt stimulated you to want to tighten that muscle tone through regular exercise.

Another phase, or course—the diet! You may discover that being on a diet may trigger some feelings inside of you that may surprise you. The American Diabetic Association diet is the most balanced diet available, and affords you much variety with the exchange program. Even so, just being on a diet and having to account for all you eat can make you angry, frustrated, or even depressed. This is why 3D provides another vital phase —some very positive input!

We believe you will be amazed at how the workbook and the teaching tapes will clarify for you what is happening inside of you emotionally. They will give you encouragement and hope as you discover more about yourself. These down-to-earth, realistic devotional aids will help you not only come face-to-face with you, but also face-to-face with the One who knows and loves you intimately.

From 3D's beginnings, God has combined the understanding of the needs of the body, mind, and spirit together in this very unique program. We in 3D are aware that He has raised up the concepts and ideas that you have been reading, and it is only with His help that any of us can even attempt to live disciplined lives.

All the suggestions that are included in these materials have been a part of 3D from the beginning days. If you find that you are only able to handle a few disciplines at a time, express this to your leaders immediately. Then agree together on the parts of the program that you are going to make a commitment to work on. Perhaps after three weeks you can add another discipline and keep taking further steps. But don't get discouraged. It is not easy to start all over in reshaping your life by learning how to eat a different way, or how to share a thought or feeling with another individual. It is not easy to sit in a circle and pray for people you hardly know. But it is possible.

Disciple-ship

Webster's Dictionary defines discipleship as one who follows his/her Master.

All 3 "D's" are integral parts of the "3D" program. They complement one another. Solomon in Ecclesiastes said that a three-fold cord is not easily broken. Let's take a brief look at how essential each "D" is to "3D"!

The first "D" in 3D is Diet. Healthy eating will after weeks and months become part of your thinking, and your way of life. Not just for three months, six months, or even a year experiment, but hopefully you will benefit from this well-balanced eating and it will be an established lifetime pattern which you enjoy.

Discipline, the second "D" is one of the tools of God to aid in the breaking of old habits and the establishing of new ones. In accepting disciplines we are propelled toward our goal. When we accept the disciplines of the 3D diet, we move closer to the goal—healthier bodies and loss of weight (if that's what we need). To reach any valuable goal, we have to learn discipline. In 2

Timothy 2, Paul speaks about three disciplined disciples—a soldier, an athlete, and a farmer. The soldier goes to boot camp and undergoes the rigors of training to be a good soldier. The athlete trains to obtain the prize, and the farmer rises early and labors hard to receive the fruit. There are no instant doctors, artists, nor instant musicians. They all require rigorous training and discipline. Whatever we practice long enough becomes part of us. Your 3D experience can provide a framework to motivate and assist the learning of personal discipline. Discipline brings liberty.

The third "D"—Discipleship—is more difficult to define. In John 15:8, Jesus says: "This is to my Father's glory, that you bear much fruit, showing yourselves to be my disciples" (NIV).

Yes, our discipleship is revealed by the fruit we bear. Through the 3D program, we trust you will discover that true spirituality is reality and honesty. That truth frees us to become well-integrated persons, healthy in body, disciplined and able to make good choices. Discipline enables us to choose long-range goals above short-range satisfactions. The disciplines empower us to follow "the Master"—Jesus. Remarkably, fruit thrives and flourishes as we obey and follow Him.

Our goal is Discipleship: following Jesus Christ through our life. Diet and Discipline are two of the ingredients of Discipleship. God extraordinarily uses them to beckon us on to Discipleship.

Resources

The devotional workbooks—*Devotions for A New Beginning* and *Devotions for Daily Living*—are required materials for a successful group. These two workbooks will give you material for one full year of the program. It is within the pages of these books that you will find the tools for discipleship. There is no other way to make this third "D" a part of your life than to study His word and give time to devotional readings and Scripture memorization. Then apply these truths to your life daily.

DEVOTIONS FOR A NEW BEGINNING
Session One: A New Beginning
Weekly Devotional Themes:
The Lordship of Christ
Why Discipline?
God's Will or My Will?
Learning to Listen
The Blessing of Obedience
Nobody Tells Me What to Do
Those Whom I Love I Reprove
If We Confess Our Sins
Emotions: What to Do With Them

When Light is Darkness
Your Mind: A Battleground
What is Discipleship?

A twelve-week session in which the Biblical concept of accountability works itself into the heart of the 3D member. Here is where you learn to take your dieting seriously. You come to grips with your specific problem—and what it is going to take to resolve it. Everyone's needs in the weight department are different, and you will follow a plan ideally suited to your need. And yet, whether you have ten pounds to lose or a hundred and ten, the key is accountability—to God, to others, and to yourself.

The workbook leads us into a knowledge of what God expects of us in very practical parts of our life. And then shows us how to bring Him into the middle of our problems. Many of us may know the answers in our heads—but have trouble applying them with all our hearts. The daily questions in the workbook will bring the head and heart together.

As we come to know what He expects of us, we become more comfortable with—and desirous of—being accountable to Him. This session also focuses on the importance of sustained prayer—to Him for help, understanding and grace, and for others in the program. For without the power of ongoing prayer any success will almost certainly be temporary and superficial.

You will be challenged to memorize one verse of Scripture each week—a verse well-chosen to help you withstand the inevitable temptations and frustrations that will be in your path on this walk.

Accountability also takes on a very practical form. You will be asked to keep an accurate and honest food diary, and to record in detail the spiritual disciplines which you have agreed to undertake. You will be amazed at what a blessed corrective such a simple act of obedience can be!

Session Two: The Heart of the Matter
Weekly Devotional Themes:
The Joy of Being Open
Learning to Forgive Yourself
The Hidden Bitter Root
Won't Somebody Love Me?
What's Wrong with Being Right?
Who, Me, Angry?
Why Doesn't Someone Understand?
The Fine Art of Getting Even
Every Day is a New Beginning
Fear: Faith in the Wrong Person—You
Playing God—The Sin of Control
Pressing Toward the Goal

By this time you will have been part of the 3D program for more than three months. You will have had success in losing weight, you'll have made long-term friends and will have come into that new dimension in your spiritual walk. You'll have learned how to care for others and will have a deeper awareness of the power of prayer.

And you'd like to think that at last the diet aspect of your need is under control.

Well, it may be, but this is the session where you learn there is still lots to learn—about maintenance, plateaus, slow weight loss, and even weight gains that slip in unnoticed. Here is where you learn the lessons that will last a lifetime.

In this twelve-week session we get down to what really motivates us in our hearts. Often we are surprised to find that it is not what we thought. Sometimes, in fact, it comes as a shock—but that is where God smiles and friends help. Learning to identify the root causes of our undisciplined behavior and calling them by name—jealousy, vindictiveness, anger, self-pity, pride, fear—can be tremendously freeing. It is often a painful process, and too frequently we avoid pain by anesthetizing ourselves with food, sleep, busyness—anything that keeps us comfortable.

Being comfortable in our Christian life can be a grave hindrance to spiritual growth. We need to know who we are—and where we need His help. For He will help us. We can change. Thousands upon thousands have undergone profound change, spiritually and mentally, as well as physically, in the 3D program.

Session Three: Pressing On
Weekly Devotional Themes:
New Lamps for Old
Learning to Live with Me
Learning to Live with Others
Learning to Live Openly
But It Hurts
Forgiving One Another
Perseverance
The Fork in the Road
Changing Habit Patterns
The Peace of God
His Mercy Endures
Where Do We Go From Here?

By now you will have become a seasoned veteran of 3D and will be learning what it means to be a Soldier of the Cross. But at this point you'll no doubt be struck with the subtle temptation to let up. Here is where so many defect and drop away. For it is precisely when we have gained a measure of success that we are most vulnerable.

Here is where so many of the 85% of successful dieters become overconfident and ultimately fail. "Frankly, I'm tired of dieting. I've lost the weight I wanted to lose, I'm praying and reading my Bible almost every day, and I simply don't have the time to keep going to meetings and filling out food sheets."

The choice will be yours. In this session the guideline is responsibility; you are now responsible for making the right choices. And that choice is to persevere. This twelve-week session challenges us to firmly root and establish the work God has done in us. And now we begin to see the fruit of our obedience overflowing into the lives whom our life touches. For the real test of what has happened in us will be how it blesses others.

But when we have been blessed spiritually—and have been a blessing to others—it is easy to neglect the basic, practical needs which drew us into the program in the first place. And so, these twelve weeks are also a time to recommit ourselves to the practical side of 3D—eating sensibly, exercising regularly, and being obedient to all the nitty-gritty disciplines which have laid such a good foundation. "It is the little foxes which spoil the vine. . . ."

Session Four: Along the King's Highway
Weekly Devotional Themes:
Baby Steps
Side Steps
Back Steps
Traps and Pitfalls
Wayward Wanderings
Road Blocks
Growing Weary on the Road
Resting Places
Heeding the Signs
Uphill, Downhill
Traveling Light
Walking with Jesus

As you have already discovered, 3D is so much more than a weight-control program! It has been teaching you to see with God's eyes—and with His compassion. As you begin to realize how little you truly know about what motivates you, you come to a new understanding of God's patience and mercy with you—of His enduring love for you.

He wants you to change, to become more conformed to the image of His Son. But He also knows that you cannot, unless you truly want to. And so, by His Spirit, He is drawing you gradually into a deeper spirituality—until ultimately, nothing is more important than pleasing Him.

This fourth devotional workbook offers key assistance on that journey. With its daily Bible readings, questions, and weekly Scripture verse to memorize, it will clarify and crystallize the progress you are making along the King's Highway. It can be used in a support group, as a church or prayer group's Bible study, or as a personal or family devotional.

If you will do each lesson faithfully for the twelve assigned weeks, they will seal what God has been showing you, so that you will easily recall them, in times of great need.

One thing: If you are willing to be transparently honest as you answer the questions, He will give you fresh insights, even as you write.

Session Five: Heart Beats
Weekly Devotional Themes:
The Examined Heart
The Troubled Heart
The Best of Rooms
The Uncommitted Heart
The Hungry Heart
A Wandering Heart
The Broken Heart
The Heart Has Its Reasons

The Steadfast Heart
A Heart Filled with Gratitude
The Awakened Heart
The Satisfied Heart

God is very interested in the condition of our hearts, physically and spiritually. He wants us to know the importance of keeping our hearts in good condition. This session helps you examine the important elements involved in having and maintaining a healthy heart. "You made us for youself, and our hearts are restless until they rest in you" (St. Augustine).

JESUS LOVES ME
DAY BY DAY DEVOTIONALS
Weekly Devotional Themes:
Jesus Loves Me, This I Know . . .
Who Is This Jesus?
Learn of Me
Tell Me the Old, Old Story
The Hidden Gospel (Old Testament)
They Testify of Me (New Testament)
Believe in Me

You may have sung it hundreds of times: "Jesus loves me." But do you really know it? Here are some new thoughts about that "unbelievable" good news. This book also explores the question: "Who is this Jesus who loves me?" As you follow these daily Bible devotions and meditate on them, you will come to know better the answer to that question. Whether in group study or as an individual devotional reading, *Jesus Loves Me* will encourage you to a livelier, more active faith-walk with Him.

My Thoughts Along the Way

This journal, interspersed with uplifting quotations, will inspire participants to record their thoughts throughout the 3D program.

Other Resources and Helps for Your Spiritual Journey

Doors into Prayer
Emilie Griffin

Acclaimed writer Emilie Griffin presents a simple and personal introduction and invitation to the life of prayer. From the earliest beginnings of prayer in childhood and in moments of stress and trouble, building gradually and gently toward a disciplined prayer life, Griffin acquaints readers with the basic fundamentals of prayer and explores the many types of prayer that believers have used through the centuries.

Surrendering to God:
Living the Covenant Prayer
Keith Beasley-Topliffe

Has prayer come to mean rote repetition? Is there hope for a deeper experience of prayer? Drawing from his own experience of praying the Covenant Prayer, a classic verbal prayer made popular by John Wesley, Rev. Beasley-Topliffe provides a brief history of the Covenant Prayer and a meditation on each phrase of the prayer, illuminating his personal experience with the words of many classic spiritual writers. Unlike many of today's books on prayer, which are either collections of written prayers or discussions of general methods and forms of prayer, this book brings new excitement and insight to a simple, yet transforming prayer that many know by heart.

Even Among These Rocks
Steven D. Purcell
Foreword by Eugene Peterson

Beginning in "The Desert of Temptation" and ending with "The Final Act" of Jesus' crucifixion, Steven Purcell, conference director at the Schloss Mittersill Centre in Austria, invites readers to journey with him through the forty days of Lent—a journey of self-discovery that ultimately reveals the staggering depths of God's love.

Purcell illuminates his spiritual reflections with the paintings of Rembrandt and Caravaggio, the poetry of T.S. Eliot and Denise Levertov, the music of Vaughan Williams, and many others, as well as his own lavish watercolor illustrations. A devotional for Lent or any time of the year, *Even Among These Rocks* is a stirring celebration of creativity infused by the Holy Spirit throughout the ages.

Relief for the Body, Renewal for the Soul
G. Scott Morris

In 1987, G. Scott Morris, a United Methodist minister and a board-certified physician, opened the doors of his medical clinic to the working poor, elderly, and homeless of Memphis, Tennessee. Today, Dr. Morris's clinic is America's largest faith-based health center for the poor. In his book, Dr. Morris recounts the true stories of twelve of his most remarkable patients. For those who doubt that there is hope for America's largest social problems, these easy-to-read, inspirational stories provide convincing proof to the contrary.

A Grief Unveiled
Gregory Floyd

With heart-breaking honesty, Gregory Floyd reveals his journey through grief after the death of his youngest son. This book is a witness to the intimate presence of Christ in the midst of unbearable loss.

ECHOES OF ETERNITY, VOLUMES I AND II
Hal M. Helms

Our oldest Christian traditions invite us to listen when we pray. The 365 meditations in each of these volumes contain Scripture verses and "impressions" of God's words for every day of the year.

THE PRACTICE OF THE PRESENCE OF GOD
Brother Lawrence
Translated by Robert J. Edmonson

The story of a jovial seventeenth-century lay brother who spent much of his monastic life in the kitchen, these simple words of wisdom teach us how to experience a daily, moment-by-moment fellowship with God.

TALKING WITH GOD
François Fénelon
Edited by Hal M. Helms

Fénelon offers sage spiritual advice on topics such as choosing friends wisely, what to do when feelings fail us, living in the present, and handling criticism.

MEDITATIONS ON THE HEART OF GOD
François Fénelon
Translated by Robert J. Edmonson

Fénelon's advice on seeking God in the midst of everyday life will encourage all who desire to know His heart.

ORDER FORM

Payable in US funds only. We accept Visa, MC, or checks. Call (800) 451-5006, fax (508) 255-5705, order Online at www.3DChristianDiet.com, or mail your orders to: Paraclete Press, PO Box 1568, Orleans, MA 02653.

SAVE 20% OFF 6 OR MORE COPIES OF ANY ONE TITLE

Resource Materials   **Price**

____ 3D by Carol Showalter/$25   _____

____ Devotions for a New Beginning/$19.95   _____

____ Devotions for Daily Living/$24.95   _____

____ Leader's Manual/$6.95   _____

____ Jesus Loves Me (Devotional Book)/$12.95   _____

____ My Thoughts Along the Way/$12.95   _____

____ Doors into Prayer/$13.95   _____

____ Surrendering to God/$13.95   _____

____ Even Among These Rocks/$22.00   _____

____ Relief for the Body, Renewal for the Soul/$13.95   _____

____ A Grief Unveiled/$13.95   _____

____ Echoes of Eternity, vol. I/$12.95   _____

____ Echoes of Eternity, vol. II/$12.95   _____

____ The Practice of the Presence of God/$9.95   _____

____ Fénelon: Talking With God/$10.95   _____

____ Fénelon: Meditations on the Heart of God/$11.95   _____

Book Total: $ _____

Subtract 20% for 6+ copies of any one title _____

5% Sales Tax (MA): $ _____

Postage & Handling: $ _____

Total Amount Due: $ _____

Shipping & Handling Charges:

Orders under $10......................$3.95   Orders $50.00–$79.99..............$7.95

Orders $10.00–$29.99..............$6.50   Orders $80.00–$124.99............$11.00

Orders $30.00–$49.99..............$6.95   Orders $125.00–$299.99..........$17.00

Bill my

Credit Card # _____ exp. _____

❏ Visa   ❏ MC

Signature: _____

Bill to: _____

Address _____

City _____ ST ____ ZIP _____

Daytime Phone _____

Ship to: _____

Address _____

City _____ ST ____ ZIP _____

Please allow 2–3 weeks for US delivery.
This offer is subject to change without notice.
Tracking code: M3D2